Coping with Diverticulitis

Overcoming Common Problems Series

Selected titles

A full list of titles is available from Sheldon Press
on our website at www.sheldonpress.co.uk

The A to Z of Eating Disorders
Emma Woolf

Autism and Asperger Syndrome in Adults
Dr Luke Beardon

Chronic Pain the Drug-free Way
Phil Sizer

Coping with Aggressive Behaviour
Dr Jane McGregor

Coping with Diverticulitis
Peter Cartwright

Coping with Headaches and Migraine
Alison Frith

Coping with the Psychological Effects of Illness
Dr Fran Smith, Dr Carina Eriksen
and Professor Robert Bor

Dementia Care: A guide
Christina Macdonald

Depression and Anxiety the Drug-free Way
Mark Greener

Depressive Illness: The curse of the strong
Dr Tim Cantopher

Dr Dawn's Guide to Sexual Health
Dr Dawn Harper

Dr Dawn's Guide to Toddler Health
Dr Dawn Harper

Dr Dawn's Guide to Your Baby's First Year
Dr Dawn Harper

Dying for a Drink: All you need to know to beat the booze
Dr Tim Cantopher

The Empathy Trap: Understanding antisocial personalities
Dr Jane McGregor and Tim McGregor

Everything Your GP Doesn't Have Time to Tell You about Alzheimer's
Dr Matt Piccaver

Everything Your GP Doesn't Have Time to Tell You about Arthritis
Dr Matt Piccaver

Gestational Diabetes: Your survival guide to diabetes in pregnancy
Dr Paul Grant

The Heart Attack Survival Guide
Mark Greener

The Holistic Guide for Cancer Survivors
Mark Greener

Hope and Healing after Stillbirth and Early Baby Loss
Professor Kevin Gournay and Dr Brenda Ashcroft

How to Stop Worrying
Dr Frank Tallis

IBS: Dietary advice to calm your gut
Alex Gazzola and Julie Thompson

Living with Angina
Dr Tom Smith

Living with Multiple Sclerosis
Mark Greener

Living with Tinnitus and Hyperacusis
Dr Laurence McKenna, Dr David Baguley
and Dr Don McFerran

Mental Health in Children and Young People: Spotting symptoms and seeking help early
Dr Sarah Vohra

The Multiple Sclerosis Diet Book
Tessa Buckley

Parenting Your Disabled Child: The first three years
Margaret Barrett

Sleep Better: The science and the myths
Professor Graham Law and Dr Shane Pascoe

Stress-related Illness
Dr Tim Cantopher

Taming the Beast Within: Understanding personality disorder
Professor Peter Tyrer

Therapy Pets: A guide
Jill Eckersley

Toxic People: Dealing with dysfunctional relationships
Dr Tim Cantopher

Treating Arthritis: The drug-free way
Margaret Hills and Christine Horner

Treating Arthritis Diet Book
Margaret Hills

Understanding Hoarding
Jo Cooke

Vertigo and Dizziness
Jaydip Ray

Wellbeing: Body confidence, health and happiness
Emma Woolf

Your Guide for the Cancer Journey: Cancer and its treatment
Mark Greener

Lists of titles in the Mindful Way and Sheldon Short Guides series are also available from Sheldon Press.

Overcoming Common Problems

Coping with Diverticulitis
Second edition

PETER CARTWRIGHT

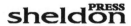

First published in 2007, second edition published 2016

This edition published by Sheldon Press in 2019
An imprint of John Murray Press
An Hachette UK company

1

A CIP catalogue record for this title is available from the British Library

Trade Paperback ISBN 9781529305043
eBook ISBN 9781847094384

Printed and bound in Great Britain by Clays Ltd, Elcograf S.p.A.

John Murray Press policy is to use papers that are natural, renewable and recyclable products and made from wood grown in sustainable forests. The logging and manufacturing processes are expected to conform to the environmental regulations of the country of origin.

Sheldon Press
Carmelite House
50 Victoria Embankment
London EC4Y 0DZ

www.sheldonpress.co.uk

Contents

Foreword

In Western countries, the prevalence of diverticular disease increased during the last century. Diverticular disease is currently one of the five most costly gastrointestinal disorders affecting the US population. This has widespread implications, as it is now one of the commonest surgical conditions encountered in the Western world. This increase probably reflects both an increase in detection and an ageing population.

Thirty years ago, the proportion dying from diverticular disease was decreasing. However, during the last 20 years annual age-standardized rates of hospital admission and surgical intervention have increased by 15 per cent, from 20.1 per 100,000 to 23.2 per 100,000, while inpatient and population mortality rates remain unchanged. This increasing burden of disease demands robust, evidence-based management guidelines. Without such data, implementing management to a growing group of people would be costly for both health care providers and patients alike. This can be a disease that can change one's life, and as such it is understandable why those with it want more information.

Such information can be difficult to find and the medical literature is confusing and contradictory in places. As our knowledge and understanding of diverticular disease and its complications improves, the concepts related to management continue to change. Much of the published literature is out of date due to better diagnostic tools, and newer therapeutic opinions.

This book presents the general consensus view of the literature as regards conservative and surgical management of diverticular disease. The aim has been to provide patients with information in a factual and detailed manner, yet in plain English that allows them to participate in the management of their problem. The management decisions are at times difficult, and the consequences significant, so patient participation is beneficial for both patient and doctor. This book is a major step in patient education and participation in the management of their disease.

Professor Frank A. Frizelle
Professor of Colorectal Surgery
Christchurch School of Medicine and Health Sciences
Christchurch
New Zealand

Acknowledgements

Although I take full responsibility for the content of this book, it is important to recognize the considerable help received from a wide range of knowledgeable people.

For commenting on a draft text, I am grateful to the following consultant gastroenterologists: Professors Derek Jewell, David Rampton, Jonathan Rhodes and Robin Spiller, and Doctors Nadeem Ahmad Afzal, Anton Emmanuel and Neil Stollman. Thanks also go to consultant surgeons Professor Neil Mortensen and Mr Geoffrey Hutchinson, consultant physician and psychotherapist Professor Nick Read and to specialist nurse Lesley Bolster.

The Diet chapter was the most difficult to prepare, and valuable guidance was given by consultant gastroenterologists Professor John Cummings and Dr Martin Eastwood, nutritional sciences lecturer Dr Kevin Whelan, and private registered dietitian Elaine Gardner.

Information and encouragement was also supplied by staff and members of the Bladder and Bowel Foundation and by members of the Colostomy Association.

Finally, many thanks to my wife, Yvonne, for her unfailing encouragement.

Note to the reader

This is not a medical book and is not intended to replace advice from your doctor. Consult your pharmacist or doctor if you believe you have any of the symptoms described, and if you think you might need medical help.

Introduction – the basics of diverticulitis

What is diverticulitis?

The purpose of this book is to provide easy-to-understand information for people who have been diagnosed with diverticular disease (DD), and for their relatives and close friends. The information is intended to provide reassurance and to help the patient feel that he or she is in greater control of their situation.

Diverticular disease refers to the appearance of small pouches (sacs), known as diverticula, that protrude outwards from the wall of the large intestine. Each diverticulum (singular of diverticula) consists of a small part of the inner lining of the intestine that has been forced through the muscular layer of the intestine forming a small hernia (balloon). It is as if the normal intestinal tube had been squeezed and the pressure had made little protrusions of it to appear through any weak points. The number of these protrusions differs between individuals, and can be one or two, or as many as several hundred. They are usually the size of small grapes (5–10 mm in diameter).

In addition to the term diverticular disease, you may also hear of diverticulosis and diverticulitis. What is the difference between these terms? The definitions used in this book are:

- diverticular disease: used to describe all forms of the presence of diverticula;
- diverticulosis: the condition in which these small sacs appear, but cause no symptoms;
- symptomatic diverticulosis: the condition in which some symptoms are experienced, but there is no infection of the sacs;

- diverticulitis: the inflammation of the sacs (caused by an infection), involving abdominal tenderness and pain and a slight temperature, and from which other complications may develop.

It is possible that your diagnosis may not tally with the definitions above. For example, you may be told that you have diverticulitis, but no infection is present. Sometimes health professionals use the term diverticulitis because the word 'disease' in the term diverticular disease might suggest to the general public that it is contagious, which it is not. Doctors and nurses may think that the patient will find diverticulitis a more acceptable term.

The majority of people with the protruding sacs have diverticulosis, with no signs or symptoms. For the minority with symptoms, the most common are abdominal pain, change in bowel habits (constipation or diarrhoea) and bleeding from the back passage.

Although diverticula can be found in any part of the intestine, they are commonly found in the large intestine, particularly in the sigmoid part of the colon. To understand the significance of this, it is useful to consider the digestive tract and the role that the large intestine plays.

The digestive tract

The digestive tract (also known as the intestine) is a tube that runs through the body from the throat to the anus. Its purpose is to convert food particles into absorbable materials and energy for the body, and to remove the unusable parts of food.

Food provides the body with molecules so that it can grow and replace worn-out cells and tissues. Food also provides energy so that all the parts of the body can work. The difficulty with food, however, is that it cannot easily be taken into the body. This is because, in addition to absorbing food molecules, the body also has to keep out harmful germs. The discrimination between food molecules and harmful germs is made by specialist (epithelial) cells. These epithelial cells fit tightly together forming a layer that lines the intestine and that controls entry from the digestive tract into the body.

The food that we eat consists mostly of carbohydrate, protein and fat, and these molecules are all too large to pass through the epithelial barrier. These large molecules need to be broken down (digested) so that they are small enough to pass through the epithelial layer and into the body.

The process of digestion starts in the mouth (see Figure 1 overleaf), where food is chewed into smaller pieces. Also in the mouth, enzymes contained in saliva start the chemical breakdown of the large food molecules. From the mouth, the food passes down a long tube (the oesophagus) into the stomach, which is where the digestive tract widens to form a bag. Here, the food is held while being churned by the stomach's rhythmic movements. Enzymes are secreted from the wall of the stomach and these break down the food molecules further. The contents of the stomach become liquefied (known as chyme) and are released into the small intestine.

The small intestine consists of three parts: the duodenum, the jejunum and the ileum. The duodenum is a short section of the intestine immediately after the stomach, into which more enzymes are secreted and where acid from the stomach is neutralized. The main part of the small intestine, the jejunum and ileum, is where the digested food (chyme) is absorbed into the body. The small intestine is about 6.5 m (22 feet) long, which allows enough distance for most of the digested food molecules to be absorbed.

The final part of the digestive tract is the large intestine, which is where diverticula usually form. The large intestine is about 1.5 m (4 feet) long, and is shorter than the small intestine. The names of the small and large intestines are due to the width or bore of the tube. In other words, the large intestine has a wider bore than the small intestine.

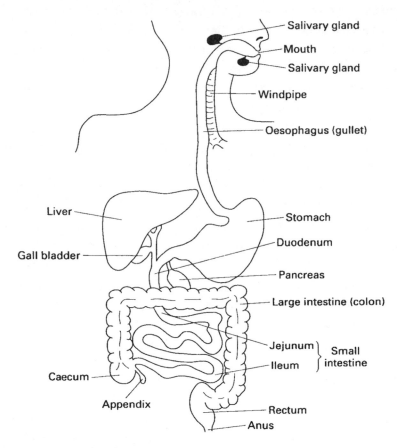

Figure 1 The digestive system

If all the digested food has been absorbed through the small intestine, what is the function of the large intestine? It used to be thought that its only purpose was to reabsorb some of the water (and salt) into the body, leading to the solidifying of the waste into faeces. These faeces, being solid, are easier to hold in the lower part of the large intestine until ready or convenient to be released.

More recently, however, the resident bacteria in the large intestine have been recognized as important. There are trillions of bacteria living in the human large intestine. They feed on the parts of food not digested by the human enzymes, including starch and other complex carbohydrates. Some of the molecules broken down by the bacteria are absorbed into the body through the wall of the large intestine rather than being used by the bacteria. These molecules can provide up to 10 per cent of our daily energy requirements.

The large intestine consists of three parts: the caecum, the colon and the rectum (see Figure 2). Diverticula may appear in any part of the colon, but in European and US populations diverticula arise mainly in the sigmoid colon. About 90 per cent of patients have diverticula in this area, and 45–65 per cent have diverticula only in this area and in no other part of the intestine. In contrast, within Asian populations diverticula are found more widely along the colon, particularly on the ascending (right-sided) colon.

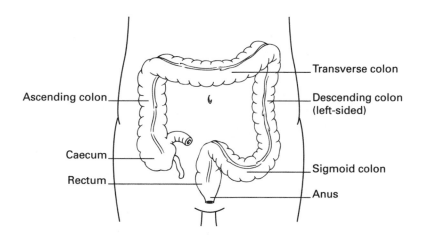

Figure 2 The large intestine

The solid part of the large intestine, as opposed to the space, is known as the colonic wall. It consists of several layers forming two main parts: the mucosa (that contains digestive and immune cells) and the muscles (that control contraction). The diverticula are formed when part of the mucosa is squeezed out through a weak point in the muscle layers.

How many people are affected?

Diverticular disease (DD) is a very common condition in Western countries (Europe and North America) among the middle-aged and older. The precise numbers with diverticula are not known, as most people have no symptoms. It is not possible to tell if a person has diverticula unless they develop symptoms or the diverticula are discovered following a medical examination for another purpose. The best estimate is that between a quarter and one-third of people over the age of 40 have diverticula, which increases to about a half of all those over 70. Diverticula are rare in people under the age of 30.

Of the large numbers of people with diverticula, the majority will, as noted, never suffer any symptoms. The exact proportion that develop symptoms is not known, mainly because the numbers with symptomatic diverticulosis are not known, due to uncertainty over diagnosis (see Chapter 3 for details). Given this uncertainty, only a rough estimate can be given of the proportion of people with diverticula who will experience symptoms, which is about 15–20 per cent.

Of those people who develop symptoms of DD, a small proportion, probably less than 5 per cent, will have a very severe form that will require emergency surgery. The great majority of people with symptoms of DD do not require emergency surgery, but if diverticulitis develops (i.e. the diverticula become infected), many can be treated successfully with antibiotics. With the diverticulitis brought under control, most people will find that their DD causes no further trouble. The evidence suggests that between two-thirds and three-quarters of people with symptoms of diverticulitis will have just one bout of such inflammation. Some research, however, shows that on occasion, individuals with diverticulitis have psychological and physical symptoms long after acute attacks. In some cases, they may develop what amounts to a form of irritable bowel syndrome (IBS), or persistent digestive problems can occur and persist after an acute bout of diverticulitis. These are striking findings which add to growing evidence that, for some, diverticulitis goes beyond isolated attacks and can lead to a chronic condition, according to work by the University of California, Los Angeles (UCLA) in 2013 and 2014.

Another type of symptom is haemorrhage (bleeding) from the back passage. This occurs in about 15 per cent of people who have symptoms arising from diverticula.

Less than a fifth of people with DD symptoms will need to enter hospital as an inpatient, and of these inpatients about 20–25 per cent will undergo surgery. Of those undergoing surgery about one-third will have complications of diverticulitis, such as perforation, abscess or fistula. These complications are explained in Chapter 3.

The figures given above for admissions and surgery are a generalization, and the proportions may be different in some hospitals due to the specific policies of the hospital and its medical staff.

Looking at the general population of Western countries, the proportion of people who will develop symptoms of DD at some time during their lives is perhaps about 5 per cent, and only about a fifth of these will need to be admitted for treatment as an inpatient. In other words, although diverticula are very common from middle age onwards, only a small proportion of people will be bothered by this condition. Sadly, acute diverticulitis, a disease traditionally seen in people older than 50, is now being seen in younger adults who are obese, according to a study conducted by the University of Maryland Medical Center's department of radiology in Baltimore, MD.

The main points of these statistics are:

- diverticulosis of the colon is a very common condition;
- less than a fifth of people with diverticulosis develop any symptoms;
- DD is more common among older people and is rare among people under 30;
- diverticulitis, without complications, is successfully brought under control by antibiotics in the great majority of cases;
- at least two-thirds of people who have an initial bout of diverticulitis will have no recurrence;
- less than a fifth of people with symptoms of DD will need to be admitted to hospital for treatment;
- of those admitted to hospital, about 20–25 per cent will require surgery.

Figure 3 opposite illustrates how only a small proportion of people with diverticula are troubled by symptoms.

The structure of the book

Chapter 1 covers the cause of diverticular disease. This is important, because an understanding of the origins of the condition and how it develops can be helpful when considering how to cope with the day-to-day challenges of DD. It may also be helpful if new treatments arise and if you want to be an active participant in discussions with your doctor.

The causes of DD are not fully understood, so the chapter considers the subject by examining the evidence and the various possible explanations. In this way you will be in a better position to reach a conclusion as to the most likely explanation.

In Chapter 2, you will find a description of the process by which the doctor decides on the diagnosis. It includes a list

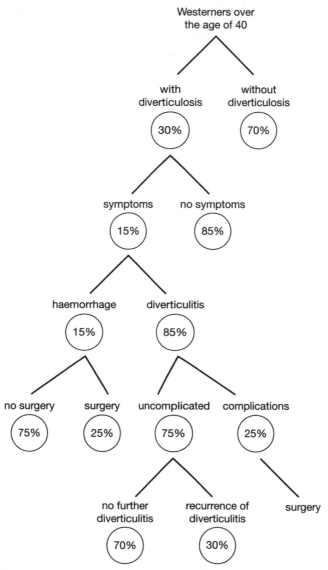

Figure 3 Frequency of different forms of DD, excluding symptomatic diverticulosis

of the different types of exploratory examinations. These tests may be used not just during diagnosis, but also during periodic check-ups or if there has been a change in symptoms. By understanding the range of investigations that the doctor can undertake or order, you will reduce the uncertainty in your mind and consequently the level of anxiety.

Chapter 3 describes the symptoms of different types of DD. This will help you to identify the type of DD you have. The chapter also describes the treatments available for each type of DD.

As Chapter 1 identifies dietary fibre as an important factor in the development of DD, Chapter 4 covers the subject of diet in some detail. The desirable amount and type of dietary fibre is described, and the types of food that are high in fibre are also covered.

If you have recurrent troubles from your DD, then dealing with the day-to-day consequences of the condition will be important. Chapter 5 covers issues relating to living with DD.

Among people who have symptoms of DD, about 5 per cent may have to undergo surgery to deal with persistent trouble. Chapter 6 describes in detail the circumstances in which surgery may be undertaken, as well as the experiences that can be expected immediately prior to and after the surgery. Unless you like to know all the possible outcomes, it may not be necessary to read this chapter until your doctor or surgeon raises the possibility of surgery.

Similarly, Chapter 7, describes all the main points about having a stoma, which only affects a small minority of people with DD. This chapter need not be read unless you expect to have a colostomy (or ileostomy). Please note that a stoma is usually temporary in people who have had one formed during surgery for DD.

Chapter 8 has the title 'Special circumstances' and covers four categories: people from East Asia, the younger patient (under

40), the immunocompromised, and differences between men and women. There are distinct characteristics in each case, and these are described in this chapter.

Chapter 9 is entitled 'Future developments'. It covers topics in which there may be substantial developments in the future. The topics are painkillers, IBS-like symptoms, aminosalicylates, probiotics, laparoscopy (key-hole surgery), maternal diet and the hunter-gatherer diet.

I do hope you find this book clear and easy to read, and that you will wish to refer to it again if the circumstances of your DD change in the future.

1

What causes diverticular disease?

In this chapter, the search for a clear understanding of the cause of DD will be described as a scientific detective puzzle, in which a picture of the cause gradually emerges. Why should you, as the reader, bother with this chapter when all you want to know is the cause?

For a patient, the value of having a good understanding of the cause of the condition is that:

- understanding gives a greater sense of control over the condition;
- knowledge places you in a better position to have a productive discussion with your doctor about treatment.

In the latter case, you might be in a position in which standard treatment has not eradicated all your symptoms. This may be the point at which you would want to discuss with your doctor why the treatment is not fully effective and to consider other treatments. A good understanding of the cause will help you in that discussion.

Evidence about the cause is given in some detail so that you can judge the matter for yourself. I do hope you find the following story fascinating. If you do not wish to go into such detail at this time, a summary is found at the end of the chapter.

Discovering the cause

Complete agreement has not yet been reached within the medical profession as to the causes of DD of the colon. Much is known, however.

When scientists and medical researchers are devising a hypothesis (an initial explanation) for a disease, they look at any peculiar characteristics that may give a clue to its cause.

Three characteristics of colonic DD are notable:

- the condition appeared only about 100 years ago;
- it is absent from rural, economically underdeveloped populations;
- it is more common in people over the age of 40.

Each of these characteristics will be looked at in turn to see what light it sheds on the cause of DD.

A new disease

Prior to the twentieth century, the presence of diverticula in the colon was so rare in people of Europe and North America that it was viewed as a medical curiosity. By the 1970s, diverticula had become common in those over the age of 40.

When precisely did DD start to increase in frequency? Although by 1920 the condition had not yet appeared in medical textbooks, the British surgeon Sir John Bland-Sutton remarked that 'During the last ten years, acute diverticulitis … is recognised with the same certainty as … appendicitis', describing it as 'a newly discovered bane of elders'. By 1930, it had been estimated that 5–10 per cent of colons in people over the age of 40 bore diverticula.

The statistics point to the disease starting to appear in noticeable numbers early in the twentieth century. What had happened in Britain at the turn of the twentieth century to cause such a development?

Incidence in different populations

The first clue in explaining the rapid rise in the number of cases of DD came from studies and reports by doctors in various parts of sub-Saharan Africa. They noticed that DD was almost non-existent among rural Africans. For example, in a large Johannesburg hospital (2,000 beds) only one case of diverticulosis was found in 2,367 autopsies from 1954 to 1956. In a teaching hospital in Lagos, Nigeria, serving a population of 400,000 people, just two cases of diverticulitis were diagnosed between 1963 and 1965.

As the intestine is affected by DD, researchers looked at the types of food consumed and found a major difference between Africans and Europeans in the amount of fibre in the diet. Dietary fibre is the part of food not digested by human enzymes within the small intestine. Comparing the weight of stool production in people from different parts of the world, it was found that on average each person in rural populations in Africa produced more than 400 grams weight of stool per day compared to 60–150 grams by Westerners. This difference in weight is explained wholly by the amount of fibre in the diet.

In the light of this information, two doctors, Painter and Burkitt (see 'Further reading'), proposed a hypothesis that DD is caused by a reduction in the amount of fibre in the diet. They argued that the key date in Britain for this change of diet was around 1880, when a new method of producing flour, roller milling, was introduced. This method produced flour with a low level of fibre, and the flour became widely used in Britain. Other factors that led to a reduced amount of fibre in the diet were increased consumption of meat and refined sugar. These items were more commonly consumed as a consequence of increased prosperity, improvements in rail and sea transport and refrigeration.

Furthermore, Painter and Burkitt pointed out that the rise in the death rate from DD was halted in Britain during and immediately after the Second World War, and started to increase again thereafter. They argued that during the war (and for a while afterwards) white bread was not available and refined sugar was strictly rationed.

Forty-year development period

If the fibre hypothesis is true, it does not follow that an unsuitable diet will cause disease immediately. The statistics show that the incidence of DD increases rapidly after the age of 40, suggesting that it usually takes 40 years of a low-fibre diet for the protrusions to appear in the intestine.

This timescale also ties in with Painter and Burkitt's theory, because 40 years after the introduction of roller milling (in 1880) takes us to 1920, the time when doctors were starting to notice the appearance of diverticula in their patients.

The hypothesis of low-fibre diet causing DD, promoted by Painter and Burkitt in the 1970s, stimulated a great deal of scientific interest. In a vigorous debate, some aspects of the hypothesis were questioned.

Low-fibre hypothesis challenged

Criticism of the low-fibre hypothesis comes in five forms:

1 There may have been no real increase in the prevalence of diverticula.
2 There may be a genetic factor in the development of diverticula.
3 There may be something in the diet, other than fibre, causing DD.
4 Lack of exercise may cause DD.
5 DD may simply be a disease of ageing.

No increase in prevalence of diverticula?

Could the dramatic rise in prevalence of DD in Western countries be more apparent than real, due to poor recognition of diverticula by nineteenth-century scientists? Supporting this suggestion are some data from the turn of the twentieth century. In a German medical journal of 1899, it was reported that the post-mortem examination of 28 colons found 18 (64 per cent) containing diverticula. A year later, in the same journal, 15 out of 40 colons (37.5 per cent) were found to contain diverticula. However, in another German journal, published in 1902, only seven colons were found to contain diverticula out of 8,133 examined.

It has been argued that such great variation in statistics may be explained by the difficulty in identifying diverticula in colons from autopsies. Alternatively, it could be argued that the two studies giving a high incidence of diverticula were based on small numbers and they may have not been typical of the population.

X-ray pictures of barium enemas (see Chapter 2) are less prone to difficulties in identifying diverticula and have given more consistent results. Five studies between 1929 and 1949 gave an incidence of diverticula ranging from 6 per cent to 12 per cent. These studies involved a total of 42,000 cases, with no study involving fewer than 2,000 cases. Barium enema studies in the second half of the twentieth century showed at least one-quarter with diverticula present in the colon.

Therefore, despite some uncertainty about the prevalence of diverticulosis at the turn of the twentieth century, the great majority of statistics show a pattern of increases in the incidence of diverticula throughout the twentieth century. It does appear that DD has become more common.

A genetic explanation?

The next criticism of the low-fibre hypothesis is that the almost complete absence of DD in black Africans might be explainable by racial/genetic factors rather than by diet.

The incidence of DD among urban black Africans is, however, increasing. A study in a South African hospital found 16 patients diagnosed with DD over a 14-month period in 1974–75, compared with no cases over a three-year period in the 1950s at the same hospital. All of the affected patients were urbanized people whose diets involved a very high intake of refined carbohydrate and a low fibre content. Consumption of fruit and vegetables was low, while meat was eaten daily. Some were in relatively well-paid employment and could afford a range of foods, while the others were domestic servants who ate the low-fibre diet of the households in which they worked.

In an urban hospital in East Africa (Nairobi, Kenya), 226 barium enemas undertaken over a two-year period in the late 1970s found 15 cases of DD.

Most convincing of all, data in the mid-1980s showed that the prevalence of DD among black Americans was the same as among white Americans.

In summary, the incidence of DD in African populations appears to increase in line with the adoption of Western diet and lifestyle. Explanations for the development of DD based on racial/genetic differences are therefore not persuasive.

A dietary explanation, but not fibre?

The third criticism of the dietary fibre hypothesis is that the rise in prevalence of DD may be due to factors in the diet other than dietary fibre. The change in fibre consumption in Western countries, as measured through official statistics, has not been as substantial as might have been expected. Measures of total fibre consumption in the USA from 1909 to 1975 show a fall of 28 per cent and data from Britain show a slow and progressive decline from 1880 to the 1970s. Consumption of cereal products and potatoes decreased substantially in both countries, but this was partly offset by an increase in (non-potato) vegetable consumption and some increase in fruit consumption.

Furthermore, it has been pointed out that as rural Africans eat more fibre than Westerners, they eat less of other items, including meat. Any of the differences in diet between these two populations might be relevant in explaining the different rates of DD.

A recent review of data from South Africa compared the diet of urban black Africans with rural Africans. The urban population's diet had more protein (13 per cent) compared with that of the rural population (10 per cent), higher fat consumption (25–30 per cent compared with 15–20 per cent), and lower carbohydrate consumption (55–65 per cent compared with 70–75 per cent). Given that DD is starting to appear in urban South Africans, these data strengthen the case for diet being a cause, but do not clarify whether increased meat and fat consumption or lower fibre consumption are the key factors.

In a study in the mid-1970s in Ghana, 16 patients with symptomatic DD had apparently changed little in their eating habits from their traditional high-roughage, low-calorie diet. The patients were all from upper social classes and it does raise the question of whether other items, such as meat, had been added to the diet.

An especially useful study in clarifying potential causes of DD is the Health Professionals Follow-up Study (HPFS). The HPFS is a continuing dietary survey of more than 47,000 US male health professionals over the age of 40. During a four-year period, 385 of the study participants were newly diagnosed with DD. From questionnaires on diet and lifestyle, and with the use of sophisticated statistical analysis, a very strong inverse relationship was found between total dietary fibre consumption and the risk of developing DD. This inverse relationship means that an increase in the consumption of dietary fibre reduces the risk of developing DD.

Other analysis of the HPFS study found that protection against DD was provided by the insoluble part of dietary fibre, particularly cellulose. More information on the sources and types of fibre can be found in Chapter 4.

The HPFS study also showed a statistically significant positive association between DD and the consumption of processed meat as well as for beef eaten as a main dish. This suggests, but does not prove, that red meat contributes to the development of diverticula.

The case for meat consumption playing a role in causing DD was further strengthened by a study in Greece in which the diet of two groups (those with and without diverticula) was compared. The study found that people with diverticulosis not only consumed significantly fewer vegetables and less brown bread, but also consumed more meat (lamb and beef).

In a study in the UK of people without symptoms of DD, consisting of 264 non-vegetarians and 56 long-standing vegetarians, diverticula were found in 33 per cent of the non-vegetarians and in only 12 per cent of the vegetarians. The former consumed on average 21 grams of fibre per day compared with 42 grams for the vegetarians. The vegetarians, therefore, consumed twice as much dietary fibre and had about one-third the rate of DD compared with the non-vegetarians. Perhaps the vegetarians were benefiting from the absence of red meat in their diet as well as from higher amounts of dietary fibre.

The way in which red meat may increase the risk of developing diverticula is unknown. One hypothesis is that bacteria in the intestine transform partially digested meat into a chemical that is harmful to the normal function of the intestinal wall.

In summary, the data on diet strongly confirm that shortage of dietary fibre is the main factor in causing DD. There is also evidence that insoluble fibre is particularly helpful in protecting against DD. Frequent consumption of red meat may also be a contributory factor to DD, although the mechanism is unknown.

A sedentary lifestyle?

The fourth criticism of the dietary fibre hypothesis is that diet might not be involved in diverticula formation at all. As rural Africans work physically much harder than Europeans, exercise could be a factor.

A study in Greece found that DD was more prevalent among people with sedentary occupations than in more active populations. Furthermore, the HPFS study, described above, shows an inverse relationship between physical activity and the risk of developing symptoms of DD. In other words, physical activity probably reduced the risk of developing DD. Most of the association was with vigorous activities such as jogging, running, cycling and racquet sports. It is not clear, however, how physical activity might have such an effect, although exercise does seem to reduce constipation. The subject of exercise is considered more fully in Chapter 5.

While lack of exercise may increase the chance of developing DD, it is not as important a factor as low fibre intake.

An effect of ageing?

Diverticula are rare in Westerners younger than 30, and the risk of developing diverticulosis increases as a person gets older. These facts prompted Painter and Burkitt to suggest that it takes about 40 years of continual low-fibre diet weakening the colonic wall before protrusions appear, and that the longer a person consumes a low-fibre diet the more likely it is that DD will develop.

An alternative explanation is that the colonic wall ages along with the person, and that the ageing process makes the formation of diverticula more likely. The increase in prevalence of DD, it is argued, was due to an increase in life expectancy during the twentieth century. With more people living longer, there are more people with older colons.

Ageing is associated with a decrease in the tensile strength of the colonic muscles. Tensile strength is a measure of how stretchy something is. The colon is less flexible the older a person becomes.

The flexibility of the colon is caused mostly by two substances, collagen and elastin, which are gel-like proteins. These proteins are found in connective tissue, which is material that holds together the cells and the layers of the colonic wall. The colonic wall is normally very stretchy and is able to expand whenever a large volume of faeces passes along the intestinal tube.

For reasons that are not clear, as a person ages collagen and elastin change their structure and cause the colon to be less flexible. This reduced stretchiness in the colonic wall appears to make a colon more likely to develop diverticula. This may be because the pressure within the colonic space is greater during movement of the faecal contents since the colonic wall resists changing shape.

While an ageing colon may be more likely to develop diverticula, is ageing the only factor? Why, for example, do diverticula appear in the middle-aged of some populations and not in the elderly of others?

One explanation is that the ageing process of the colon appears to be accelerated by a low-fibre diet. For example, in a study of two groups of rats receiving either a low-fibre or a high-fibre diet, it was found that the collagen in the intestines of the low-fibre rats (that developed diverticula) had deteriorated in a way similar to the ageing process. In other words, a low-fibre diet seemed to make the colonic wall less flexible, and this was associated with the development of diverticula. Also, detailed examination of human colons from autopsy found that collagen structure was 'older' in people with diverticula than in those without, making the colon more rigid.

Furthermore, a characteristic of most colons with diverticula is a change in the form of the muscles of the colonic wall. This includes alteration to elastin, the other major component of connective tissue. In the longitudinal muscle of the colon of people with DD, there is a much greater amount of elastin present and this has the effect of shortening the longitudinal muscle and creating more pronounced haustra (compartments) along the colon. This in turn is likely to increase pressure within the colonic space.

The prevalence of DD within Western populations increased during the twentieth century, which throws light on the role of ageing in the cause of DD. A study in north-east Scotland of the number of people admitted into hospital with DD showed an 84 per cent increase over ten years (1958–61 to 1968–71). In northern Finland, the number of people admitted into a hospital with severe diverticulitis rose by 58 per cent over a 15-year period (1986–2000).

However, in a similar study in England over ten years (1989–90 to 1999–2000), the increase in the proportion of elderly people in the population during that decade was taken into account. By making such an adjustment to the statistics, the increase in hospital admissions for DD was a more modest 12 per cent. This increase is a lot less than that recorded in the first two studies above, and suggests that a major factor in the growth in prevalence of DD is the increase in the proportion of older people in Western populations. However, ageing of the population is not the only factor in explaining the continuing rise in the number of people affected by DD.

In summary, ageing of the colon is clearly a factor in the development of DD. It is not clear, however, which is more important: premature ageing of the colon promoted by low-fibre diet; or the natural ageing that occurs from middle-age onwards.

Conclusions on the criticisms

Having considered criticisms of the Painter and Burkitt hypothesis on low-fibre diet, it is clear that the low-fibre explanation remains intact and that it is the strongest explanation for the development of diverticula, along with the ageing of the colonic wall.

This conclusion is supported by a number of studies involving laboratory animals, such as rats, rabbits and monkeys. The studies consistently showed that a low-fibre diet was associated with the development of diverticula and high pressure within the colon. The opposite was true for a high-fibre diet.

Furthermore, a study in England of DD patients with a matched group without DD, found that those with diverticula consumed half the amount of cellulose in their usual diet, compared with the DD-free group. And in another British study, 58 people with symptomatic DD were found to have in their usual diet an average fibre intake of 15 grams per day, which is one-third less than the average for the general public.

How might a low-fibre diet cause diverticula?

By what mechanism might a shortage of fibre in the diet cause the appearance of diverticula? An explanation is found in the way that the colon is structured and how it moves the contents.

The semi-liquid faeces in the colon are moved by muscle contractions of the colon, without any conscious control by the person whose colon it is. Furthermore, such movements usually occur without the person being aware of them. These involuntary muscular contractions are of a wide variety, but the majority are associated with contractions of segments of the colon.

These segmental contractions of the large intestine have the function of improving absorption into the body of two items: water from the faeces, and energy-providing molecules (fatty acids) arising from bacterial breakdown (fermentation) of large undigested food molecules. In order to maximize the amount of water absorption and fermentation products, the faeces are mixed in backwards and forwards movements over short distances, so that they remain in the same general area of the colon. Consequently, it takes a relatively long time (about two days) for faeces to travel the four-foot length of the large intestine.

The segments of the colon are called haustra (singular: haustrum) and are a few centimetres long. The haustra are bordered and formed by narrow, shallow indentations called haustral markings that are found around the outer surface of the colon. The haustral markings are formed by a slight constriction of the circular muscle of the colon and are the points at which muscle contraction most often occurs in moving colonic contents.

Contraction of the circular muscle of a haustral marking causes a haustrum to become more distinct and to reduce in size. This contraction moves the contents in either direction, depending on the behaviour of the neighbouring haustrum. Several adjacent segments may contract in sequence so that the contents are pushed in a particular direction; or segments may contract independently so that the contents move backwards and forwards, causing mixing of the faeces.

With a high-fibre diet, the colon expands to a wide diameter to hold the large volume of faeces. It is thought that, with a larger bore to the colon, the haustral marking contraction enters less far into the colonic space. This produces less internal pressure, because there is a larger opening connecting with the neighbouring haustrum. In comparison, a narrow-bore colon arising from a low-fibre diet will contract so that each haustrum almost closes the colonic space, causing increased pressure. The extra pressure within the colonic space is eventually released by forcing the inner lining of the colonic wall out through the muscular part of the wall, forming a diverticulum.

Another possible factor in the formation of diverticula relates to the muscles of the colonic wall. The circular muscles thicken and the longitudinal muscles shorten, perhaps as a consequence of straining to move small-volume faeces. The muscle changes accentuate the segmentation of the colon, so that it becomes concertina-like in shape and the space within the colon is filled with many folds of the inner lining. The muscle changes are common in people with DD and are seen when colons are starting to show signs of producing diverticula. It can be assumed that the severely segmented and narrowed colon is much more likely to produce high internal pressures when muscle contractions take place.

Diverticula protrusions appear between strands of the longitudinal muscle and usually where a small artery enters the circular muscle of the colon. This is a point of weakness in the colonic muscle (see Figure 4).

It is believed that the protrusions appear initially at the time of contraction and disappear afterwards, but if this process is repeated often enough, the protrusions become permanent diverticula.

This suggested mechanism for the formation of diverticula is supported by consistent evidence of greater pressure within the space of the colon in people with DD. Also, several small studies on people with DD found reduced colonic pressure after treatment with a high-fibre supplement.

Some people are naturally more prone to constipation than others, perhaps due to the way that their intestinal muscle contractions function. Constipation is the production of hard pellet-like stools that are hard to excrete. People who are prone to constipation, irrespective of the amount of fibre consumed, are also likely to be prone to developing diverticula, according to the explanation given above.

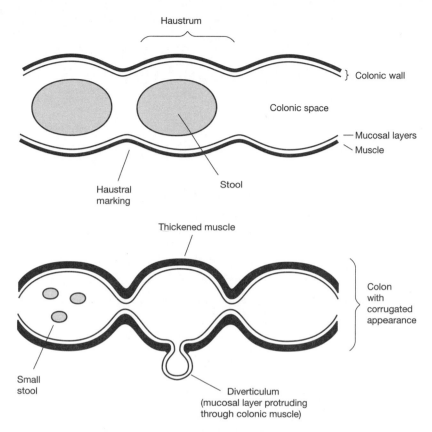

Figure 4 Comparison of a normal colon and a diverticulum-forming colon

In conclusion, the consensus among specialists is that DD is caused by the consumption of low-fibre diets, and that diverticula are more likely to appear in people with inflexible colonic walls, usually caused by an ageing process. Those who frequently consume red meat and who take little exercise may further increase the risk of developing DD.

2

Diagnosis and tests

The symptoms of DD that most commonly cause a person to visit their family doctor are:

- abdominal pain;
- bleeding out of the back passage;
- change in bowel habits (frequency of going to the toilet).

These symptoms are similar to those caused by a number of other illnesses, and this is why your family doctor is likely to refer you to a hospital doctor specializing in gastrointestinal disease.

Case history

The first thing a specialist doctor will do is ask questions about the symptoms. The doctor will want you to describe what is wrong, in your own words. This can create a problem – how to talk clearly about your bowels, and without feeling embarrassed.

Saying you have an 'upset tummy' or 'stomach trouble' will not be enough. The doctor will want to know more precisely what you mean by this. It is therefore worth planning how you will describe the symptoms. How will you describe bodily waste? Liquid excreted from the bladder is formally known as urine, but is also referred to as 'No. 1', 'pee' or 'piss'. These words are reasonably acceptable in public, but what should you use to describe the solid waste? The words 'No. 2', 'poo', 'shit', 'faeces' or 'stool' are all options for getting your point across to the doctor. What about describing the process of passing the solid waste? While doctors may use 'defecation' when talking among themselves, 'passing stools', 'opening one's bowels' or 'having a bowel motion/movement' might be more comfortable alternatives for you. The more slang-like 'having a crap/shit' could also be used.

There is also the difficulty of describing the part of the body involved. The word 'bottom', like the word 'tummy', is a bit vague. There may be no alternative but to use the technical terms of 'anus' and 'rectum'. However, 'back passage' is frequently used to describe both anus and rectum together.

Whatever words you use, please remember that doctors are very unlikely to be embarrassed. They have heard it all before! The most important point to remember is to describe your symptoms as accurately as possible. Don't leave something out just because describing it may make you embarrassed. Your health is far more important than a bit of social discomfort.

If speaking about bowels is really too embarrassing, you could write everything down in a note to give to your doctor.

The symptoms that your doctor may be most interested in are:

- the type of abdominal pain (e.g. occasional or continuous, cramping or steady, sharp or dull, where in the abdomen, whether relieved by defecation);
- the frequency with which you pass stools;
- what your stools look like;
- whether any blood is passed.

The doctor may also be interested in whether you have experienced fever or weight loss. Furthermore, the doctor may ask whether you feel that something specific started the symptoms, if these symptoms have occurred before, and whether any of your relatives have suffered similar symptoms.

Initial physical examination

After speaking to you about your symptoms and taking your past history, the doctor will usually make a manual examination of your abdomen by pressing different parts to see if there is any tenderness or hard lumps. The doctor may also make a digital examination of your rectum. This involves your lying on your side and the doctor, wearing a lubricated thin plastic glove, putting a finger into the rectum through the anus. The doctor will be feeling for any abnormal shape.

The most common tests used when investigating symptoms that may be of DD are:

- contrast enema;
- endoscopy;
- computerized tomography (CT scan).

All of them require the intestine to be cleaned of all faeces, although a CT scan can be of value, in some circumstances, without bowel cleansing.

Bowel cleansing

It is important to clear the colon of all faeces for several reasons:

- to make it easier to assess the state of the large intestine and achieve accurate diagnosis;
- to reduce the risk of perforation of the bowel by the endoscope (currently occurring in fewer than one in 500 cases);
- to shorten the time taken to complete an endoscopy and, if relevant, the length of time the patient is sedated.

The process of cleaning the bowel is often referred to, by doctors and nurses, as 'bowel preparation' or 'prep'. The term bowel preparation is also used for the product used to clean the intestine. There are several different ones that may be used for bowel cleansing and you will be given written instructions on how to undertake the process.

In most cases, a powder is added to water and this is drunk a day or two before the test. The cleanser will cause diarrhoea and you can expect to visit the toilet frequently. As you will have to clean your bottom many times, you may consider adult wet wipes or water spray to clean yourself, if there is a risk of the skin around the anus becoming sore. There are also creams for nappy/diaper rash that may be helpful.

After taking the cleansing product you will probably only be allowed a clear fluid diet until the test has been completed. A clear fluid diet includes clear juices without pulp (e.g. apple, grape), clear soups, jelly, ice lollies, clear hard sweets, tea or coffee without milk and soft drinks; in fact, any food you can see through at room temperature. The only exception is red coloured fluids that may discolour intestinal secretions and be mistaken for blood. Certain medications, such as iron preparations, may also be stopped to help ensure a clear view.

One of the purposes of a clear fluid diet is to provide sufficient liquid to counteract the loss through diarrhoea and so overcome the risk of dehydration. You are likely to feel hungry with this diet as it does not provide sufficient calories and nutrients for daily needs. This is why it is advisable not to continue a clear fluid diet for longer than five continuous days.

For a day or two before taking the cleanser product, you may be advised to follow a low-residue diet in order to reduce the volume of waste in the large intestine that needs to be cleared out. The hospital staff will provide you with a low-residue diet to follow, which will exclude all high-fibre foods and supplements.

It is important to follow the instructions for the cleansing product carefully, because if your bowel has not been cleaned properly, the doctor (or specially trained nurse) may cancel the procedure and ask you to return on another occasion.

Contrast enema

A contrast enema involves the use of an x-ray machine. X-rays are a type of energy, in the form of waves, that can penetrate most substances. When x-rays are aimed at a human body, most will pass through, but some will hit parts of the body that are radio-opaque (i.e. they stop most x-rays from passing through). An x-ray machine contains an x-ray film, which is light-coloured and turns dark when hit by those x-rays that have passed through the body. Differences in the amount of x-ray that reaches the film create an image (known as a radiograph or radiogram) that can be examined and interpreted by a doctor.

While a radiograph can provide an image of the abdomen, it is not particularly good at visualizing soft tissue organs. To overcome this problem, liquids known as 'contrast media' have been developed. A contrast medium blocks the passage of x-rays through the body and creates an image on the radiograph that distinguishes between the organ to be diagnosed and the surrounding tissue.

A contrast enema is a liquid that is inserted into the back passage. The patient is asked to lie down on his or her side, facing away from the doctor or nurse. A lubricated tube is inserted into the rectum, and to ease entry the patient is asked to use their anal muscles to bear down as if to defecate. A bag containing the enema liquid is held above the patient's body and the liquid is allowed to flow slowly along the tube into the rectum.

When the enema has been delivered, the tube is removed gently by the nurse, who then applies light pressure over the anus with toilet tissue or a gauze pad. The patient is asked to tighten his/her anal muscles to help hold in the enema liquid.

The enema liquid will be at body temperature to reduce the tendency of colonic muscles to expel it. It is likely that there will be some involuntary colonic muscle contractions in response to the insertion of the enema, and this may cause some spasmodic pain. The radiographer, the person who takes an x-ray picture, will ask the patient to move into different positions so that the liquid coats as much of the large intestine as possible.

The most commonly used contrast medium contains a substance called barium sulphate. The barium medium is of a chalky texture. It is radio-opaque, and as x-rays are passed through the body, the presence of the barium sulphate creates a clear image of the shape of the large intestine. If diverticula are present then some of them will appear on the image. However, some diverticula fail to fill with the barium liquid and their presence will not be identified. A better image is usually obtained if a small amount of air is pumped into the barium-lined colon. This is known as a 'double-contrast' enema.

There are several drawbacks with barium enema. It can sometimes be a strain to excrete the barium liquid, and any that remains in the intestine can promote constipation. Also, if the barium contrast leaks into the abdominal cavity through a perforation of the gut wall there is a danger of peritonitis developing, although this is a very rare occurrence. Furthermore, on completion of the enema process the bowel has to cleaned again if either of the other two main tests are to be undertaken. Therefore, although the barium enema method gives a good picture of diverticula, it may take place after an endoscopy or a CT scan rather than before.

Water-soluble contrast media (e.g. gastrografin) are also used. Iodine is the radio-opaque substance, and the contrast liquid is used either as a drink (a 'swallow') or as an enema. It does not cause harm if it leaks through a perforation, because in time it will be absorbed. Therefore, it tends to be used in more severe cases of suspected DD, or after surgery. In the case of the intestine being obstructed, it might help to free the obstruction by increasing the water flow through the narrowing. A drawback with water-soluble contrast is that it does not coat the intestine as well as barium contrast. For some people, it can be a challenge to keep the enema from leaking out of the back passage; more so than with barium contrast.

Even if diverticula are identified on a radiograph, other tests may take place. This is because diverticula are very common in people over the age of 50 and yet in the majority of cases they cause no symptoms. Therefore, the symptoms of which the patient complains may be caused by another disease and the doctor needs to make sure that the diagnosis is accurate.

Endoscopy

Endoscopy is another test that can be used to investigate the cause of abdominal symptoms. An endoscope is an instrument that allows a doctor to view the interior of the digestive tract. It consists of a flexible tube with a light at one end and an eyepiece at the other. Endoscopes are available in various lengths, and are usually inserted through the mouth or the anus. In the case of investigations into suspected DD, the tube is inserted into the large intestine via the anus and is manipulated so that the doctor can see different parts of the large intestine.

There are different types of endoscope. The one most commonly used in investigating suspected DD is a sigmoidoscope. This is of two types: the rigid and the flexible. The flexible sigmoidoscope can view further into the large intestine than the rigid one, and can reach as far as the descending colon. As the areas most commonly affected by DD in Europeans are the sigmoid and descending colon, the doctor can learn more about the diverticula, particularly whether any of them are the source of any bleeding.

Another type of endoscope is the colonoscope, which is long enough to travel the whole length of the large intestine. It is used particularly if a bleeding diverticulum needs to be identified and it is not in the left side of the colon. Modern colonoscopes have a video camera that allows the doctor to look at the colon on a monitor rather than through an eyepiece, and take a video recording of the colon. It is also possible from the tip of the colonoscope to release water and air, the former for washing waste (so that it can be sucked up) and the latter to widen the space in the colonic tube. A consequence of having pressurized air added to the colon is that some of it will escape out of the anus. This should not be resisted. It is normal and should not be a source of embarrassment. Feeling an urge to have a bowel movement is also a common experience during a colonoscopy. The whole colonoscopic procedure usually takes about half an hour, but may take longer. It may therefore be worth considering passing urine before entering the endoscope room to avoid discomfort from a full bladder.

There is an increased risk of perforating the bowel wall if the endoscope tube mistakenly enters a diverticulum and pressurized air is used. All staff who undertake endoscopies are highly trained and will be aware of the risk.

In addition to viewing an image of the large intestine, an endoscope can also take small samples from the bowel wall for examination under the microscope. This is painless as the lining of the intestine does not contain nerves that feel pain. Microscopic examination of tissue is a way of checking whether there are any abnormalities to the mucosa (inner layer of the intestinal wall) such as cancerous cells or signs of inflammatory bowel disease, both of which are possible explanations for some of the abdominal symptoms. It should be noted that people with DD are not more prone to cancer of the colon than the rest of the population.

An endoscopy is often performed by a gastroenterologist (a doctor who specializes in the digestive system) or by a specially trained endoscopy nurse. The patient will have to take off most of their clothes and will be given a hospital gown to wear. A mild sedative may be given to relax the patient, especially if it is a colonoscopy. The patient will be asked to lie on their side with knees drawn up toward the abdomen. The doctor will gently insert a gloved finger into the anus to check for tenderness or blockage. Then the thin, well-lubricated tube is inserted and moved forward as the doctor views the lining of the colon.

It will take 1–2 hours for the sedative medication to wear off, before going home. It may be helpful to have a friend present when the doctor or nurse gives instructions on being discharged, and to accompany you home. It is dangerous to drive or use machinery for 12–24 hours. Bloating or crampy gas pains may be experienced after the test, and if a biopsy was taken there may be traces of blood in the stool for a few days.

Computerized tomography (CT scan)

If the diverticula look extensive or if the symptoms are diverse or severe, a CT scan may be undertaken as it is less invasive than an enema or an endoscopy. Furthermore, CT scan pictures show more of the internal structure of the abdomen, compared with a contrast enema radiograph. The CT scanner is also useful in identifying any complications of diverticulitis, such as a fistula or an abscess.

Unlike the contrast enema that produces a simple picture of the whole length of the colon, or the endoscope that gives images of the inside of the intestine, the CT scan produces a series of images of cross sections (layers) of tissue. These cross-sectional images can also be combined by the computer to give a 3-D picture.

The patient lies down on a table, is not required to change position, and moves through the hole of a large doughnut-shaped machine. The patient is asked to hold his or her breath, and a series of images are prepared by computer, based on x-ray readings.

If air is added to the colon before undertaking a CT scan,

the image is usually improved. Doctors refer to this as 'virtual colonoscopy'. The CT scan image can also be enhanced if a small quantity of contrast medium is injected into a vein.

Other tests

There are other tests that may take place, either during the initial diagnosis or at a later date when symptoms have changed. The tests include:

- blood tests;
- ultrasound scan (sonography);
- MRI scan;
- angiogram.

A sample of blood, usually taken from an arm, will be tested in a laboratory for evidence of infection. If an infection is found, this may suggest that one or more of the diverticula are infected, but it might imply another cause for the symptoms.

Ultrasound scanning (sonography) is used occasionally in DD investigations, particularly in more complicated cases, as it is non-invasive. It can be especially helpful in identifying abscesses, although the image does need careful and experienced analysis. Sonography also appears to be useful in confirming the diagnosis of right-sided DD.

In ultrasound scanning, high frequency sound waves (that cannot be heard by humans) are pulsed into the body by a smooth-surfaced hand-held gadget, known as a transducer. The sound waves echo back from tissue and blood and are received by the transducer and turned into video images displayed on a monitor beside the patient. The patient lies on a hospital bed or examining table and may occasionally be asked to change position to give a better picture. To improve the quality of the image, a cool gel is applied to the skin where the transducer is placed. The gel is wiped off at the end of the examination. The transducer gives a slight sensation of vibration on the skin. No bowel preparation is required.

Another scanning method that may be used is the magnetic resonance imaging (MRI) scanner. An MRI scanner is a tube-shaped machine in which the patient lies. The machine is noisy and it can feel somewhat claustrophobic. The MRI scanner uses magnets and radio waves to produce an image. It is good at identifying diverticula and may be helpful in pinpointing the position of an abscess or a fistula. Currently, the MRI machine is used only rarely in DD, but it is likely to be used more frequently in future.

An angiogram may help in identifying the source of bleeding. This process involves injecting contrast material to the arteries that supply the colon. The contrast medium will be shown on an x-ray film escaping from the broken blood vessel.

This description of all the various tests and investigations may seem somewhat daunting, but most people with DD will only experience a few of them. While some of the tests may be uncomfortable, none of them are painful (except on very rare occasions).

Diagnosis made

The hospital doctor will continue with tests until he or she is able to make a diagnosis with confidence. This may take some time, because although diverticula may be relatively easy to identify, it is not easy to decide whether they are the cause of the patient's symptoms or whether some other condition is to blame.

Once a diagnosis of DD is made, the condition may be monitored periodically. It is important to co-operate with your doctor when additional tests are suggested. While DD is a disease of minor symptoms for the great majority of people, complications can develop and the signs of this can sometimes appear very suddenly. By helping your doctor to be fully informed of the current state of your DD, you are less likely to experience a sudden and unexpected deterioration in your condition. This, in turn, should give you greater peace of mind.

3

Symptoms and treatments

Assuming that the diagnosis you have been given is diverticular disease, the type of DD will determine the treatment offered you.

The nature of diverticula in the large intestine varies from person to person, both in numbers and size of diverticula, and in the different parts of the large intestine affected. There may also be complications, such as infection of a diverticulum or the development of an abscess. For ease of understanding, doctors use simple categories to describe the different degrees of severity of the disease, although currently there is no unanimity on classifying the different forms of DD. It might therefore be worth clarifying with your doctor what is meant when he or she gives your diagnosis as diverticular disease or diverticulitis. Where, how many and how extensive are your diverticula? And are there any complications?

For the sake of consistency, the classification used in this book is as described in the introductory chapter. It is important to remember that these groupings are generalizations. In each individual there may be variations in symptoms that don't fit exactly or neatly into these categories.

The symptoms and treatments of DD are described under these headings:

- diverticulosis (diverticula present, but no symptoms);
- symptomatic diverticulosis (symptoms present, but no signs of infection);
- diverticulitis (infection and inflammation of a diverticulum);

- complications of diverticulitis (abscess, phlegmon, fistula, obstruction, perforation);
- haemorrhage (bleeding).

Diverticulosis

As there are no symptoms in diverticulosis, its presence is discovered incidentally to a medical examination for some other purpose. For example, you may have had abdominal symptoms, caused by another illness, which warranted contrast tests that disclosed the presence of diverticula. Or you may have been invited to undergo a colonoscopy as part of a screening programme for colorectal cancer.

The presence of diverticula can only be classified as diverticulosis if it is clear that they cause no symptoms. If there is more than one intestinal problem, it is not always easy to find out whether the diverticula are contributing to the symptoms.

Assuming that diverticulosis has been confirmed, it should be noted that there is no evidence that a diverticulum, once formed, can be reduced or removed except by surgery. On the other hand, for the majority of people diverticula cause no symptoms for the whole of their lives.

Many doctors will take the view that, as there are no symptoms, diverticulosis requires no treatment. Other doctors believe that treatment for diverticulosis should be focused on reducing the likelihood of symptoms developing. Evidence from the HPFS study (mentioned in Chapter 1) suggests that insoluble fibre, especially cellulose, acts as a preventative against developing symptomatic DD. Furthermore, the American Dietetic Association and other authoritative bodies recommend an increase in the intake of fruit and vegetable fibre to provide a range of health benefits.

There is also some evidence suggesting that red meat consumption may be a factor in the development of symptoms in DD. It should be noted, however, that the evidence for meat being a causal factor is much weaker than the evidence for a low-fibre diet causing DD.

If you have diverticulosis and you have not been given specific dietary advice, it may be worth requesting guidance from a registered dietitian, with a view to increasing the amount of fibre in your diet.

The HPFS study also pointed to exercise as having a protective effect against the development of symptoms, and therefore an increase in your physical activity may help prevent symptoms developing on from diverticulosis.

As age is associated with the development of DD, is it inevitable that the risk of symptoms will increase as a person gets older? There is no clear answer to this, but there is some evidence to suggest that not everyone's diverticula get worse over time. In a study of people with DD over a period of five years, 72 per cent showed no change in the number or size of their diverticula.

In summary, the incidental discovery of diverticulosis should not be seen as a cause for concern. The great majority of people with diverticulosis will never be bothered by any symptoms arising from this condition. Other than ensuring that you have a reasonable amount of fibre in your diet (see Chapter 4), you should try to forget about the condition, and concentrate on other matters.

Symptomatic diverticulosis

Symptomatic diverticulosis refers to people who have diverticula with symptoms, but without diverticulitis, its complications or haemorrhage.

There is a debate over the nature of symptomatic diverticulosis as to whether it is really related to DD or whether the symptoms are a form of irritable bowel syndrome (IBS), another intestinal condition. While some doctors believe the symptoms are straightforward IBS and that the presence of diverticula is merely an irrelevant coincidence, other doctors believe the IBS-like symptoms are caused by a process linked to the presence of the diverticula.

The prevalence of symptomatic diverticulosis is not known because of the difficulty of diagnosis. In a study of 128 patients admitted into hospital with a diagnosis of 'diverticulitis', 15 per cent of them were described as having diverticula without inflammation or other complication, on the basis of CT scanning (see Chapter 2). In addition, there may be other people with symptoms that are not sufficiently severe to warrant admission into hospital, but that may be symptomatic diverticulosis.

The most common symptom of symptomatic diverticulosis is pain, which can take various forms and be experienced in different parts of the abdomen. The most common pain is of a cramping/colicky type, in which the muscles of the intestine seem to be in spasm (contracting severely). The pain is usually short-lived (2–5 hours) and is most often found in the lower-left area of the abdomen.

Other symptoms of symptomatic diverticulosis are bloating and/or flatulence (passing of gas out of the back passage), the passing of mucus in the stool and a feeling of incomplete emptying of the bowels. Changed bowel habits of constipation or diarrhoea (or both) occur in some people with symptomatic diverticulosis. The symptoms of pain and bloating tend to be worsened by eating food, and relieved by the passage of flatus (gas) or stool (often pellet-like).

The treatment for symptomatic diverticulosis tends to be standard treatment for IBS, with fibre supplements, specific painkillers, anti-spasmodic drugs and, in some cases, psychological therapy.

Some patients with symptomatic diverticulosis have symptoms that are unlike IBS. Instead of being sharp and spasmodic, the pain is low-level and constant. If such pain is causing great distress to the patient then the section of the colon affected by DD may be surgically removed. Surgeons are, however, reluctant to operate when the cause of pain is unclear. One study of treatment of such symptoms, described as 'smouldering DD', showed a good outcome from surgery, with three-quarters of patients having all their symptoms eliminated.

Due to the debate over the cause of symptoms in symptomatic DD, there is a wide range of responses from doctors. If you find yourself with such symptoms, it is important to have a careful and considered discussion with your doctor so that any treatment and its consequences are based on your particular circumstances.

A fuller consideration of symptomatic diverticulosis can be found in Chapter 9, under the heading 'IBS-like symptoms'.

Diverticulitis

Up to one-fifth of people with diverticulosis will experience symptoms arising from their diverticula at some point during their lives. A common cause of symptoms is diverticulitis, which is the inflammation of one or more diverticulum. Usually just one diverticulum is inflamed, although there may be as many as four. Inflammation is a defence response by the body to the growth in numbers of a harmful microscopic living creature, usually a bacterium.

The way in which diverticulitis develops is not known for certain, but the most likely explanation is that faeces become trapped within a diverticulum. Bacteria within the faeces grow in number causing an infection, and the body's defence mechanism produces an inflammation of the diverticulum. The infection may spread to surrounding tissues, because solidified faeces in the neck of the diverticulum may rub against the intestinal wall when colonic muscle contractions take place.

Infection and the associated inflammation occur mostly in the sigmoid colon. This is partly because diverticula are usually more common in that area, but also because diverticula in the sigmoid colon tend to have narrow necks. The narrow necks increase the likelihood that faeces will lodge there and infection develop. In comparison, diverticula that occur on the right side of the colon are less likely to develop infection. They have wider necks and the faeces are more liquid, making it less likely that faeces will become trapped in a diverticulum.

The main symptom of diverticulitis is pain, usually in the lower-left abdomen, although in patients from East Asia the pain might be in the lower-right abdomen, as right-sided DD is more common in that population. The pain of diverticulitis tends to be acute and constant rather than spasmodic. Such pain may last for several days, interfere with normal daily activities, and will usually force the patient to seek medical advice. A change in bowel habits, such as diarrhoea or constipation, is another common symptom of diverticulitis. The patient is also likely to have a mild fever, and sometimes nausea and vomiting.

Blood tests usually show a rise in the white blood cell count. White blood cells are part of the immune system and an increase from their usual number is a sign that there is an infection that the body is resisting.

Standard treatment of diverticulitis is bed rest and antibiotics, and it has a high level of success in overcoming the infection. The types of antibiotic used are broad-spectrum (killing a wide range of bacteria), and poorly absorbable so that most of the drug is available to work on the intestine. The antibiotic is taken by mouth for 7–10 days. The doctor may also recommend bowel rest, which means the replacement of solid food with a clear liquid diet. The antibiotics should reduce symptoms after two or three days, and solid food may be reintroduced gradually, initially low-fibre and later high-fibre.

A person with diverticulitis may be treated either as a hospital inpatient or as an out-patient, depending on the severity of symptoms and the history of the disease. Inpatients may be treated with intravenous fluids and intravenous antibiotics.

While most hospitalized patients will respond to treatment, an estimated 20–25 per cent will require surgery during that admission. Details of surgery are found in Chapter 6. If antibiotics and bowel rest are effective in getting infection under control, the doctor will probably recommend a full examination of the colon to check that there are not any other intestinal problems.

Between two-thirds and three-quarters of patients will have no further symptoms, after an initial attack of acute diverticulitis. If, however, there is a subsequent bout of diverticulitis, the risk of further bouts thereafter is increased. With each new flare-up of diverticulitis there is a risk of complications developing, such as an abscess or a fistula. Many doctors recommend surgical removal of the affected part of the bowel after two attacks of diverticulitis, as a preventative against more serious developments. This recommendation is discussed more fully in Chapter 6 on 'Surgery'.

As with the treatment of pain in symptomatic DD, pain in diverticulitis must be treated with care as some painkillers increase the risk of complications developing. Further details on painkillers are found in Chapter 9 on 'Future developments'.

Complications of diverticulitis

The use of antibiotics and bowel rest is effective in ending the inflammation and associated symptoms of diverticulitis in at least 70 per cent of cases. If this treatment does not work or only works temporarily, then the continued inflammation may lead to a number of complications:

- an abscess;
- an inflammatory mass (phlegmon);

- a fistula;
- bowel obstruction;
- perforation of the bowel wall.

Abscess

The most common complication of diverticulitis is the formation of an abscess. An abscess is a cavity within body tissue containing pus and surrounded by inflamed tissue. Pus is a creamy viscous liquid that is the remains of a battle in the tissues between bacteria and the body's immune defence system. It consists mostly of white blood cells, plus some bacteria. Most of the white blood cells and the bacteria are dead. An abscess can be sore and tender, because the pus puts pressure on the cavity holding the pus as well as the surrounding tissues.

An abscess may arise from an infected diverticulum if the infection spreads to neighbouring tissue. One may also form if a diverticulum perforates, but rather than entering the abdominal space, the released diverticular contents become walled off.

A sign that an abscess is present is a tender lump that may be felt on pressing the abdomen. There may also be persistent fever despite antibiotic treatment for diverticulitis, and blood tests will show a high level of white blood cells (that are fighting an infection).

Some abscesses may resolve without treatment, possibly by the pus draining into the colonic space. This is particularly the case with abscesses smaller than 5 cm in diameter. Those small abscesses that do not resolve by themselves are treated with continued antibiotics and bowel rest. Larger and persistent abscesses may be treated by drainage of the pus, which should reduce pain and bring the inflammation under control. Drainage can be done if the abscess is near the surface of the skin, and involves a minor surgical operation in which a tube is inserted through the abdominal wall. To help locate the abscess, a CT scan (or sometimes an ultrasound scan) can be used.

Drainage of an abscess may occasionally be a wholly effective treatment, but is usually a temporary improvement, to be followed by an operation to cut away the abscess, along with the length of colon with which it is associated.

If abscesses are left untreated they may burst. As pus contains some living bacteria, a dangerous infection may develop within the sterile abdominal cavity.

Inflammatory mass (phlegmon)

A phlegmon is similar to an abscess, in that it consists of pus, but rather than being within a contained cavity, the pus is found in many small pockets spread within tissue that becomes a hardened mass of infection and inflammation. A phlegmon may be felt as a tender lump by manual examination of the abdomen.

In addition to being tender, an inflammatory mass is potentially painful. There is also a risk that the tissue may adhere to a neighbouring piece of intestine. Such an adhesion may cause the intestine to kink and become blocked, which in turn may lead to vomiting. There may also be pain as food is forced through the narrow intestine.

The inflammation from a phlegmon (and from an abscess) may cause irritation to the bladder, causing uncomfortable and more frequent urination.

Like an abscess, a phlegmon may have to be removed by surgery if it does not respond to antibiotic treatment.

Fistula

Rather than bursting open, abscesses associated with diverticula may on rare occasions form fistulas. A fistula is an abnormal tube or passage within the body, between an internal organ and the body surface or between two internal organs.

In the case of diverticulitis, a fistula may develop from any part of the inflamed colon. If a fistula forms it is usually between the colon and the bladder. It is formed in a gradual process in which the surface of the abscess is broken and the leaking pus is quickly enclosed by tissue, forming a protruding tube. The process is repeated many times and the tube, containing pus, gradually extends until it reaches another hollow organ or the skin surface. On completion of the fistula, the tube remains open releasing pus.

If a fistula forms between a colonic abscess and the bladder, then pus or faeces or gas may appear in the urine. Faeces may pass along the fistula, depending on the position of its starting point. Infection of the urinary tract may occur.

Colon–bladder fistulas are more common in men, probably because in women the uterus acts as a barrier to the bladder. Women may, however, develop fistulas from the colon to the vagina, particularly if they have had a previous hysterectomy. Fistulas may also connect with the small intestine, or with the skin surface.

The main treatment for a fistula is an operation to remove the section of the colon on which the fistula is found. The small hole in the organ to which the other end of the fistula was connected will usually close of it own accord, but a larger hole may need to be sewn in order to close it.

Bowel obstruction

Rarely, in about 2 per cent of patients with diverticulitis, the intestine becomes obstructed. Obstruction does not usually mean complete blockage. Rather, the intestinal tube narrows so that large lumps of food cannot pass, but liquid food can dribble through. The problem with blocked food is that, while the lumps may gradually be broken down by digestive enzymes and by churning from muscle contractions, the static food may encourage the overgrowth of bacteria, which may lead to a harmful infection.

A blockage in the large intestine may be caused by inflammation swelling the tissues surrounding the colon, and consequently narrowing the colonic space. Similarly, an abscess may compress the colon. The small intestine may also be affected by obstruction arising from diverticulitis. This usually happens when a part of the small intestine becomes kinked or twisted on being incorporated into an inflammatory mass in the area of the sigmoid colon.

Signs of obstruction include abdominal pain, bloating and vomiting. The place of obstruction may be identified by an x-ray.

The usual treatment for obstruction is to have a liquid diet or intravenous fluids. In most cases, the obstruction is temporary and will resolve as the inflammation is brought under control by antibiotics. If there are several obstructions or they are persistent, then surgery may be necessary to remove the affected area, or a tube or balloon can be inserted to widen the colon.

Perforation of the bowel wall

A diverticulum may perforate (form a tiny hole) and allow some of the contents of the colon into the abdominal space. Perforation is a rare occurrence, but when it occurs it is dangerous because it may cause peritonitis. The bursting of an abscess is another way peritonitis can occur.

Peritonitis is inflammation of the peritoneum triggered by its infection by bacteria. The peritoneum is a membrane that lines the whole abdominal space and also the contained organs.

If peritonitis develops, an emergency operation is required. The main sign of peritonitis is severe abdominal pain, often developing suddenly.

The risk of perforation is one of the reasons why it is important to treat diverticulitis as soon as possible. The inflammation increases the likelihood of perforation, due to increased pressures and distortions within the colon and surrounding tissues. Risk of perforation is also a reason why a colonoscopy is avoided in people with extensive and/or inflamed diverticula.

Haemorrhage

A dramatic symptom of DD is haemorrhage, which is the loss of a large volume of blood from the back passage. It occurs in about 15 per cent of people who have symptoms of DD. The precise cause is not clear, but it is known that a blood vessel normally present in the colonic wall becomes stretched over the dome of the diverticulum as the protrusion forms. It is this blood vessel that ruptures during haemorrhage, either at the dome or at the neck of the diverticulum.

The reason for the rupture is uncertain, but it may be that faeces trapped and hardened in the diverticulum rub against the inner wall of the diverticulum as the colon moves by muscle contractions. This rubbing process may gradually wear the blood vessel near to the diverticulum.

People who have right-sided diverticula have a greater likelihood of haemorrhage than those with left-sided diverticula. The diverticula on the right side of the colon have wider necks and domes and the blood vessel is exposed to potential injury over a greater length. Also, the bowel wall is thinner on the right side compared with the left side. These are possible explanations of why right-sided diverticula blood vessels are more prone to rupture.

Haemorrhage usually occurs when there is no inflammation and sometimes is the first sign of DD. If a copious amount of blood is released it can be very worrying to the person affected, not least because it usually comes without warning. Irrespective of the amount of bleeding, it is rarely painful.

Haemorrhage usually leads to admission into hospital for bed rest and close monitoring. It is treated initially by giving the patient plenty of fluids, including blood transfusions, to replace the loss through bleeding. In three-quarters of patients, the bleeding stops of its own accord and in about two-thirds of cases there is no recurrence. If bleeding continues, the source of bleeding is identified by means of an angiogram (see Chapter 2). When bleeding has ceased, the intestine may be cleaned with a bowel preparation to enable examination of the large intestine by colonoscope. This usually helps to confirm the site of the bleeding or to discover whether there is another explanation for the haemorrhage. Furthermore, it may be possible to stop recurrence of diverticular bleeding by the use of a tool within the colonoscope that cauterizes (seals) the wound. Persistent bleeding will probably require surgery.

Certain painkillers are suspected of increasing the risk of bleeding from diverticula (explained more fully in Chapter 9).

Conclusion

In this description of the various symptoms and treatments for different types of DD, it is important to remember that the majority of people with diverticula have no symptoms at all, and that among those with symptoms, most find there is no recurrence after the first treatment.

4

Diet

The most likely causes of DD are a low-fibre diet and the ageing of the colonic wall. Of these two factors, there is little firm information on preventing the ageing of the large intestine, although it is possible that increasing the volume of the stools in the colon, through increased fibre consumption, may hold back intestinal ageing.

This chapter will concentrate on dietary fibre, looking at:

- whether high-fibre diets reduce symptoms of DD and prevent them from coming back;
- the nature of dietary fibre;
- altering one's diet to increase the amount of fibre consumed.

Do fibre treatments work?

Is there any evidence that increasing consumption of dietary fibre reduces the symptoms of DD? In 15 studies, most but not all showed substantial benefit to patients with DD who were placed on high-fibre diets or supplements. The benefits were the reduction of symptoms and/or the prevention of symptom recurrence.

Despite these benefits, there is no evidence that diverticula will reverse and disappear. The diverticula are permanent, unless the affected section of the colon is surgically removed. Most of the colonic muscle changes are probably also permanent.

An increase of fibre in the diet is therefore unlikely to be completely effective, as the existing diverticula always have the potential for developing symptoms by infection or haemorrhage. Dietary fibre may, however, give the following benefits:

- reduce the risk of perforation of a diverticulum caused by high pressure in the colon;
- reduce the risk of haemorrhage, as there should be less movement and friction against the colonic blood vessels;
- reduce the shortening of colonic longitudinal muscles by changing the elastin from a contracted state to a relaxed state.

These mechanisms of improvement are theoretical rather than proven. They are included as a possible explanation of how increased dietary fibre consumption is likely to have some, but not necessarily complete, benefit for people with symptoms of DD. Furthermore, it should be noted that there is some evidence that long-term consumption of extra fibre (for at least three months) has an increasingly positive effect, although it is not clear why.

Changed attitudes to dietary fibre

In the light of the 15 studies reported above, it is now standard medical practice to advise patients with DD to follow a diet high in fibre. The only exception to this rule is if inflammation of diverticula is present or if the patient is recovering from surgery, when a low-fibre diet is followed (see Chapter 3 on 'Symptoms and treatments').

Prior to the 1970s, the medical profession recommended that dietary fibre in the diet should be kept to a minimum in people with DD, on the grounds that symptoms would be worsened by physical irritation of the colon. In those days, dietary fibre was known as 'roughage' and the name reflects the opinion that dietary fibre was a potential irritant to the digestive tract.

During the second half of the twentieth century, it became clear that, rather than being undesirable, dietary fibre did in fact have health benefits for everyone. There are various types and sources of dietary fibre, and to develop a dietary pattern that will help to keep your DD under control it is important to understand what dietary fibre consists of and its various characteristics.

What is dietary fibre?

In general terms, dietary fibre is the part of food that is not broken down by the body's digestive enzymes and therefore not absorbed from the human small intestine into the body. There are almost no undigestible parts of meat and therefore dietary fibre is viewed as being only present in plant materials.

Dietary fibre is classified in two main ways:

- the types of molecules;
- the effect on the intestine.

Types of molecules

The first approach points out that most of the non-digestible substances in plants are carbohydrates, which are constructed of sugar molecules linked together into a long chain. There is, however, disagreement as to which types of carbohydrate should be included in the definition of dietary fibre. Everyone agrees that molecules called 'non-starch carbohydrates' (NSCs) should be included. They constitute a major part of the walls of the cells in plants, and the cell walls give strength and structure to the plants. The main NSCs are pectin, hemicelluloses and cellulose.

The other main type of carbohydrate found in plants is starch, and this is used by the plant mainly as an energy store. Most starch is not included in the definition of dietary fibre, as it is digested by human enzymes in the small intestine. There is some starch, in certain forms, that resists digestion and arrives intact in the large intestine. This is known as 'resistant starch' (RS), and as RS does appear to have an effect on the way the large intestine functions, some people believe it should be viewed as a type of dietary fibre. Other scientists believe that only plant cell-wall material should be included in the definition.

A further complication in the definition of dietary fibre is the woody material called lignin. This is included in some fibre definitions as it is often very closely associated with NSCs in cell walls and it is not digested in humans. Lignin is not a carbohydrate, however, and some scientists do not view it as dietary fibre.

Those who favour strict molecular definitions of fibre may do so because they want to undertake carefully controlled laboratory experiments on the physical and chemical properties of these molecules. Others prefer to define dietary fibre according to the effect it has on the intestine. This latter group tends to classify fibre as 'soluble' or 'insoluble'.

Effect on the intestine

Soluble fibre dissolves in water and forms a gel, while insoluble fibre absorbs water and increases in bulk. These two types of fibre have different effects on the intestine and on health. For example, soluble fibre has been shown to be beneficial for people with diabetes mellitus and in reducing cholesterol in the bloodstream.

The HPFS study, described in Chapter 1, which found that a high-fibre diet protects against the development of DD, also found that insoluble fibre provides greater protection than soluble fibre.

There are two problems with defining fibre as either soluble or insoluble. First, not all soluble fibres are gel-like and not all insoluble fibres increase faecal bulk. The other problem is that soluble and insoluble fibres are present in all types of food derived from plants and they tend to be very closely associated and integrated. In other words, while insoluble fibre may be of greater benefit for people with DD than soluble fibre, in practice it is not easy to select foods according to those categories. It is easier to focus on increasing the total amount of fibre in the diet rather than be too concerned about what type of fibre it is.

How to increase the amount of fibre in the diet

Any change to your diet should be undertaken within a framework of healthy eating. If fibre in the diet is increased, but the overall diet is unbalanced and unhealthy, then you may have your diverticular problems relieved only to find other health problems developing through a poor diet.

What is a 'healthy diet'? This means eating a mixture of the main food types so that the body gets nutrition to meet all its requirements. In the UK the recommended healthy diet is described in the Eatwell Guide, which is represented in picture form. In the United States there is a similar government-promoted healthy eating plate.

The Eatwell Guide recommends keeping hydrated and describes five food groups. These are listed below, in order of quantity recommended, with the largest first:

- grain foods, such as bread, cereal, rice and pasta;
- vegetables and fruits;
- beans, pulses, fish, eggs, meat and other proteins;
- milk and dairy products;
- unsaturated oils and spreads.

Fats, oils, sugar and sweets are consumed in large quantities by many Westerners, although they should be consumed in small quantities. Also, meat is consumed in higher quantities than recommended, while vegetables and fruits are underconsumed. Furthermore, the grain foods that should be supplying a large proportion of the required dietary fibre are failing to do so as most products are made from refined grains from which the bran layer is removed.

If you are able to increase the amount of grain foods, vegetables and fruits in your diet, at the expense of the other food groups, not only will you eat more healthily, but you will also automatically increase the amount of dietary fibre consumed.

Which foods contain the most fibre?

Within the framework of a healthy balance of the main food types, people with DD will be looking to eat those specific foods that are high in fibre. Some of these are listed in the box below.

	High-fibre foods
Grain (cereal) products	Whole grain wheat, rice and corn (maize) products, such as bran flakes, shredded wheat, brown rice and wholemeal bread. Other grains are oats, millet, barley, sorghum and rye.
Fruits	Avocado, apricots and unpeeled apples and pears.
Vegetables	Cabbage, broccoli, Brussel sprouts, cauliflower, carrots, celery, pumpkin, sweetcorn, spinach, asparagus stems and baked potato with skin.
Legumes (peas and beans)	Almost all types of legume, including garden peas, French beans, kidney beans and baked beans.
Nuts	All nuts, especially almonds and peanuts.

There is an advantage to eating whole foods, as listed above, rather than high-fibre supplements such as wheat bran. This is because whole foods contain:

- various major nutrients in addition to fibre;
- micronutrients (e.g. minerals and vitamins) and non-nutritive components (e.g. antioxidants, phytoestrogens) that may give additional health benefits.

It is advisable to increase the amount of fibre in your diet gradually, in order to control the amount of extra gas produced within the large intestine. This is discussed later in the chapter.

It is also important to ensure that the amount of fluids drunk is increased in line with the increased fibre consumed.

Registered dietitians work within the National Health Service and you could ask to see one for guidance on developing a high-fibre diet suitable for a person with DD. There are also private registered dietitians available. You could show this chapter to the dietitian who, while highly trained, may not be a specialist in DD.

How much extra fibre?

Not all Western countries agree on the desirable amount of fibre intake for a healthily working intestine. This disagreement is caused by two factors:

- differences in the definition of dietary fibre (e.g. whether it includes lignin and/or resistant starch);
- different laboratory methods used to calculate the amount of fibre in foods (which produce different figures for the same amount and type of food).

It is therefore not possible to give a specific figure for the daily target for fibre consumption that will make sense in all Western countries.

Most Western countries do, however, conclude that their populations as a whole need to increase fibre consumption by approximately 50 per cent. People with DD may need to increase their fibre intake by even more because they tend to have less fibre than average in their usual diet, and are more likely to have colons that are relatively inflexible. Some people may therefore need to double their dietary fibre intake.

It should be remembered, however, that each individual is different and a person's usual diet may contain more or less fibre than average.

Considering fibre supplements

Although there are very good reasons to increase fibre consumption through the incorporation of high-fibre foods within the diet, there are two main reasons why fibre supplements might also be considered:

- it may prove difficult to alter one's usual eating habits to introduce high-fibre foods;
- the required increase of fibre in the diet is large, and supplements contain more concentrated fibre than foods.

Altering one's eating habits

For decades Western governments have promoted a well-balanced diet to their citizens to aid their health (see the Eatwell Guide referred to earlier in this chapter). The public has, however, tended to resist acting upon such advice. Several explanations can be given for this:

- the availability of fast foods and pre-processed foods make it easy to eat unhealthily;
- fast-paced lifestyles are not conducive to time-consuming preparation of fresh food;
- patterns of eating are established in childhood and such patterns are hard to break;
- people have developed a taste for low-fibre foods.

If people tend to be resistant to altering their usual pattern of eating, people with DD may similarly find it difficult to change to a high-fibre diet.

The quantity of extra fibre required

As explained earlier, it may be necessary for people with DD to increase the amount of fibre in their diet by 50–100 per cent. Such an increase involves not only a major change in the pattern of your diet, but also a very large increase in the quantity of fibre consumed. This is not very easy to achieve as, on average, plant foods contain only about 2 per cent dietary fibre. This compares with wheat bran, one of the main high-fibre supplements, which contains about 40 per cent fibre.

Naturally, if a person has been feeling very ill from symptoms of DD there will be a strong incentive to adopt a diet conducive to keeping the condition under control. But many people will still find it difficult to alter their eating routines substantially. In such circumstances high-fibre supplements can be very helpful.

Types of fibre supplements

Ispaghula husk

There are various types of high-fibre supplement and one that is frequently prescribed by doctors is ispaghula husk. Ispaghula is the common name for a small green plant, the proper name of which is *Plantago psyllium*. It is the husks (outer layer) of the seeds of *Plantago psyllium* that are ground to powder and used in products known as 'bulk-forming laxatives'. Ispaghula husk is also known as psyllium husk, based on the name of the plant species.

The powdered ispaghula husk is added to water and drunk immediately. Clear instructions will be on the pack. The husk powder absorbs water and forms a gel-like substance. It is important to drink plenty of water with this and other bulk-forming supplements.

Ispaghula husk is very high in fibre, and its gel-like nature shows that it contains predominantly soluble fibre. It might seem somewhat surprising that ispaghula is prescribed for people with DD despite the evidence that it is insoluble fibre that is more beneficial. However, about one-quarter of the fibre in ispaghula/psyllium products is insoluble, so there is still benefit.

Two small studies on people with DD found a significant increase in colonic pressure with ispaghula husk, when the goal should be to reduce colonic pressure. There is, however, some evidence of ispaghula husk improving symptoms of DD.

Wheat bran

Unlike the seeds of ispaghula, wheat seeds have no husk. They do have bran, which is also high-fibre and is a more integral part of the seed. During the normal milling of wheat for flour, the wheat bran is removed from the seed. This bran is 40 per cent fibre, of which almost all is insoluble.

Not all forms of wheat bran have the same benefit for people with DD. Consumption of large-particled coarse bran has been shown to reduce significantly the pressure in the colons of people with DD, but consumption of small-particled fine bran has not. This difference is probably due to the greater bulk formed in the colon by coarse bran, due to a smaller proportion of the bran being digested by gut bacteria.

Other fibre supplements

In addition to wheat bran, there are other supplements high in insoluble fibre and resistant to digestion by gut bacteria. Pure cellulose may be available as a supplement product. Even less of it is digested by human and bacterial enzymes than is bran (about 7 per cent).

Polycarbophil is a synthetic type of dietary fibre that has properties similar to those of insoluble fibre. It acts as a bulking agent, and is unaffected by bacterial degradation. There are no studies on its effect on DD.

Methylcellulose is a semi-synthetic soluble fibre that does not undergo bacterial fermentation. A small number of studies of people with DD using this substance have been undertaken and have given some indication of benefit, particularly for constipation.

Are there any disadvantages to high-fibre diets?

The following areas of potential disadvantage of high-fibre diets are considered:

- effect on bowel habit;
- inflammation;
- gas production;
- mineral and vitamin absorption;
- weight gain;
- maximum amounts consumable;
- palatability.

Effect on bowel habit

All high-fibre diets have the effect of speeding up the passage of food along the intestine – transit time – in people with constipation. This is a desirable outcome as transit times of between 40 and 50 hours tend to produce soft, well-formed stools that are excreted without straining, while people with slow transit times, of 90 hours or more, tend to have small hard stools that are a struggle to excrete.

Among people with DD who also have constipation, bran supplements have shown consistently to reduce transit time. Such people are, however, a minority among those with DD. The best figures available indicate that constipation is experienced by about 15 per cent of people with symptoms of DD.

In fact, most people with symptoms of DD have transit times that are normal, or slightly faster than normal. For them, is there any danger that the consumption of a high-fibre diet might accelerate transit time such that diarrhoea is caused?

The most clear-cut evidence on this matter is available from studies involving bran supplementation. In three studies of people without digestive complaints, it was found that those with slow transit times achieved substantially accelerated passage of faeces on consumption of wheat bran supplements.

The average initial transit time in the three studies was 94 hours, and this was reduced to 51 hours. However, in those people with fast transit times the wheat bran supplement had the effect of slowing the passage of faeces (from 26 hours to 42 hours). In other words, wheat bran supplementation had the extraordinary effect of overcoming both constipation and diarrhoea.

The method by which this occurs is not clear, but it may be that the bulk formed by bran stimulates the colonic muscles to increase their contractions in people with constipation, while in people with diarrhoea the cellulose fibre in bran absorbs some of the excess fluid and the more solid faeces flow less quickly than liquid faeces.

One study of people with DD has also shown this desirable characteristic of bran supplement. It seems likely, therefore, that there is little risk of diarrhoea developing as a consequence of consuming large amounts of bran supplements. This is also likely to be true for high-fibre whole foods.

Inflammation

A high-fibre diet is not recommended if a person has active diverticulitis or one or more of its complications. This approach is based on feedback from patients, many of whom have reported painful symptoms on consuming a high-fibre diet. It is not known exactly why dietary fibre appears to worsen the inflammation of a diverticulum and its surrounding area, but it may be that bulky faeces irritate the sensitive and tender inflamed area.

If you are consuming a high-fibre diet and you feel that a diverticulitis flare-up is starting, it may be sensible to reduce the amount of fibre you are consuming until the infection has been brought under control.

Gas production

On adopting a high-fibre diet, many people find that they have a problem with bloating or flatulence. The extra gas is caused by gas-producing bacteria in the colon breaking down some of the fibre carbohydrates. This problem usually declines or disappears after two or three weeks, possibly due to an increase in the numbers of non-gas-producing bacteria.

If you are likely to find bloating especially uncomfortable, the increase in fibre consumption should be undertaken gradually over several weeks until the desired quantity of fibre consumption has been reached.

Mineral and vitamin absorption

It has been suggested that the intake of very large quantities of high-fibre foods may deprive the body of certain minerals and vitamins, with the potential for causing disease. In theory, this might happen by attachment of minerals and vitamins to fibre stopping their absorption into the body. Well-designed human studies have not, however, shown any significant malabsorption or deficiency. There may be a small reduction in the absorption of these micronutrients, but this should not be of concern to most people, because Western diets usually contain more than enough minerals and vitamins for most people.

Some elderly people, however, do not eat a lot of food or do not have a balanced diet. As a consequence, they may be consuming relatively low levels of minerals and vitamins. In those situations, elderly people who adopt a high-fibre diet may need to consider taking vitamin and mineral supplements under the guidance of their doctor.

Weight gain

For people who are underweight there may be some additional benefit in consuming high-fibre whole foods. Such foods, particularly the soluble fibre content, will be fermented by the intestinal bacteria and be transformed into nutrients of benefit to the body. The extra nutrients provided may slightly increase a person's weight.

In contrast, people who are overweight might be concerned that dietary fibre will make them more overweight. If there is such an effect it is likely to be relatively small. This is because dietary fibre bulks out food and the extra bulk causes it to be held longer in the stomach. In turn, a full stomach tends to reduce feelings of hunger and therefore may discourage overeating.

If weight gain is experienced, it may be worth considering increasing the proportion of bran in the high-fibre diet. Compared with high-fibre whole foods, a smaller proportion of bran is digested by gut bacteria and therefore fewer nutrients are absorbed into the body through the large intestine.

Weight gain ought not therefore be a particular worry when consuming dietary fibre.

Maximum amounts consumable

Given that bran supplements are a very concentrated form of fibre, is there a danger of consuming more dietary fibre than the intestine can hold?

Food takes only about five hours to travel through the stomach and the small intestine, but the time spent in the large intestine is about ten times as long. Therefore it is the large intestine that is the important organ in coping with bran-supplemented diet. The large intestine appears to be wide and flexible enough to hold a much larger amount of faeces than is currently carried in the intestines of most Westerners. This is indicated by the fact that while Europeans pass stools weighing about 100 grams in total per day, rural Africans pass stools of more than 400 grams per day.

The main point that needs to be remembered when consuming high-fibre supplements is that plenty of fluids (2–3 litres a day) should be drunk so that the fibre becomes soft and can travel easily through the intestine.

Palatability

One of the main difficulties with coarse bran is that many people do not find it has a pleasant feel in the mouth. This may be overcome by consuming bran tablets or, if loose bran is used, it can be mixed into breakfast cereals, fruit juices or soups.

If you find that coarse bran is not tolerable, please note that fine bran, which is more palatable, still has a substantial effect in bulking faeces (about one-fifth less than coarse bran).

Another palatable way of substantially increasing insoluble fibre in the diet is to include cooked bran (e.g. All-Bran), which can be added to high-fibre breakfast cereals such as branflakes and shredded wheat. Cooked bran is more palatable than uncooked bran, but it has less of a bulking effect.

Conclusion

Your doctor is likely to recommend a high-fibre diet and prescribe a high-fibre supplement to help keep your DD under control. If you are having difficulties in following the diet, do ask for guidance and support from a registered dietitian. It should be possible for your doctor to refer you to such a professional.

Pending the adoption of a specific high-fibre diet, a simple way of immediately increasing the amount of fibre consumed is to add a handful of bran to your breakfast cereal and to eat an apple and an orange each day.

5

Living with diverticular disease

The time spent with doctors, nurses and other health profes-sionals for your DD, as well as time spent as a hospital inpatient, is a tiny proportion of your life. Most of the time you will be living by yourself or with your spouse or partner, family and close friends. It may, therefore, be worthwhile spending a little time considering how you may deal with your DD in day-to-day life.

Severity of the condition

The way in which you deal with DD will be affected by the severity of the condition. The categories that will be considered are:

- diverticulosis;
- single bout of diverticulitis;
- recurrent symptoms without a hospital stay;
- former inpatient without surgery;
- surgery undertaken.

Diverticulosis

If you have diverticulosis, discovered incidentally during a medical test for another illness, there is no need to be especially concerned about the diverticula on your colon. The great majority of people with diverticulosis will live out their lives never being bothered by symptoms of DD.

You could increase the amount of fibre in your diet and take more exercise; these changes should increase the likelihood that you will never experience symptoms of DD. Other than those changes, you can forget completely about DD and carry on with your life.

Single bout of diverticulitis

The same advice could apply to those people who have had just one bout of diverticulitis that was brought under control, and who have had no flare-ups since. As described in the introductory chapter, people who experience just a single bout of diverticulitis constitute between two-thirds and three-quarters of all people who have any symptoms of DD. Furthermore, about 90 per cent of all recurrences happen within the first five years after an attack. Therefore, if you have had just a single bout of diverticulitis and this was more than five years ago, you can be reassured that the likelihood of further trouble is very low. Just to be sure, however, do try to keep a high level of fibre in your diet.

Recurrent symptoms without a hospital stay

If you have persistent or recurrent symptoms, but they have not been sufficiently severe to cause you to be admitted to hospital for treatment, you will face more challenges in dealing with your DD compared with the categories above.

You may have been prescribed antibiotics to bring a mild form of diverticulitis under control, and you may have undergone various tests. Your doctor may have advised you to increase the fibre in your diet and to contact him or her again if the symptoms become substantially worse or change in character. But other than that, your doctor will probably have little guidance to give. You will be left pretty much on your own to deal with the symptoms and their consequences.

Further information is, however, provided in this book, in Chapter 3 on 'Symptoms and treatments', especially the section on symptomatic diverticulosis. Also, there is useful information on dietary fibre in Chapter 4.

Former inpatient without surgery

If you have been a hospital inpatient, your DD will have been quite severe. Not only is there likely to have been diverticulitis, but there may also have been related complications such as an abscess or a mass of inflamed tissue. About a quarter of people admitted into hospital for severe DD will have a surgical operation. Those that are released from hospital without any surgery may have to face the question of surgery in the future.

Different surgeons have different policies, but many will advise their patients to choose surgery after two bouts of severe diverticulitis. Surgery that takes place after careful discussion between patient and surgeon is known as 'elective surgery'. This can be quite a dilemma for the patient. While most people would want to avoid surgery if possible, the more times severe DD symptoms occur the greater the risk of complications such as abscess, fistula or perforation of a diverticulum (see Chapter 3).

There is no simple answer to the question of elective surgery. Factors involved will include the strength of opinion of the surgeon and the degree of discomfort caused to the patient by the symptoms of DD. Further information on elective surgery as well as a description of the experience before and after surgery, can be found in Chapter 6 on 'Surgery'.

Not all surgery for DD is elective. Sometimes the symptoms are so severe that a person is rushed into hospital for an emergency operation. This is usually when there has been a perforation, which is causing a serious infection with continual pain and a high temperature. It is not uncommon for the first appearance of symptoms of DD to be of this kind. This can be quite a shock to the patient who has had no obvious warning signs and is possibly unaware that he or she has any diverticula.

Surgery undertaken

If you have already had surgery to remove a section of your large intestine, you may have a stoma opening onto your abdomen. A stoma is formed by the intestine being brought to the surface of the body through a surgically-made hole in the skin. The contents of the intestine are excreted through the stoma opening, rather than through the anus, and the faeces are collected in a bag.

In surgery for DD, the formation of a stoma is usually temporary, and is intended to rest the part of the intestine near to where the damaged intestine (containing diverticula) has been cut away. It can take a while to get used to a stoma, which is discussed in Chapter 7 on 'Living with a stoma'.

In most cases, the removal of the damaged intestine also removes the cause of symptoms. Without symptoms, you can forget about DD and enjoy the relief from pain. If your doctor has seen a small number of diverticula on other parts of the intestine, you may need to continue with a high-fibre diet to reduce the chance that these other diverticula might cause symptoms in the future.

Unfortunately, in a minority of cases (about 10 per cent) the surgery does not remove symptoms completely. The cause of such continuing symptoms is not fully understood. It may be that the symptoms are like those of symptomatic diverticulosis (IBS-like), which are discussed in Chapter 3 on 'Symptoms and treatments'.

Coping with continuing symptoms

If you are unlucky and have symptoms of DD, it may be worth considering about ways of coping. Three commonly used methods are:

- carrying on with life as if nothing has changed;
- talking with friends and loved ones;
- learning everything possible about the disease.

You may have a different approach, or a combination of those listed above. Whatever your preferred method of coping, do consider whether this method is a positive choice rather than just the usual way you deal with difficulties. The difference here is that DD may be with you for a long time (unless you have surgery). A successful coping strategy for the long term may need more conscious thought.

If you carry on as if nothing has changed, others may admire your stoicism and treat you with increased respect. You will also have the comforting thought that you are not being a burden to others. However, people may underestimate the degree to which DD can disrupt your life, perhaps because they are used to bowel problems being minor and temporary. Also, over time, the demands of the DD symptoms may become greater. If things become too much for you, it might be worth considering using other strategies as well. You may, for example, find that talking to someone is helpful. Is your reluctance to talk about your worries because you have had very little practice of doing so in the past? Or is it because you fear that the person you speak to may have less respect for you? There is much to be said for the stoical approach, but do make sure that you adopt it because it suits your personality and beliefs, rather than because it is the only approach you know.

For those who enjoy talking with their friends, the benefits of conversation are patently obvious. Worries that can buzz around inside the head making one anxious can dissipate with a sympathetic heart-to-heart talk. Having someone acknowledge that you are distressed and that your worries are not unreasonable can be comforting. Also, by sharing your personal concerns you are indirectly telling the listener that he or she is important to you and is needed, which is a comfort to the person concerned. There are disadvantages to this approach, however. First, it may be difficult to find friends who are willing to listen to and discuss bowel problems. Also, if you talk too much about your illness and its consequences, you may place too much of a burden on your friend and threaten your friendship. There is also the risk that talking about a problem can sometimes become an alternative to doing something about it. You might wish to consider whether you can carry more of the burden yourself and learn more about the disease so that there are fewer unknowns to make you anxious.

The third main strategy, of learning about the condition, has the advantage that you may be reassured that you are fully aware of any imminent 'breakthrough' treatments. And in knowing about the disease you will be able to speak more confidently with your doctor. This can be particularly useful if you are having trouble with your treatment and want to talk about possible changes, or if a major decision such as surgery has to be made. Furthermore, if there are alternative therapies that look promising, you can investigate and discuss them with your doctor. The disadvantage with the learning strategy is that it can sometimes be used as an excuse for not facing up to the day-to-day problems caused by the disease. By desperately holding out for a cure, you may delay the process of accepting the condition and adapting to it.

If adjusting to this recurrent condition is proving difficult, you could discuss with your doctor whether there are any psychological or counselling services available that may help you. If you are religious, you will know that prayer is a powerful aid.

Close relationships

Those who love you will react in various ways to your illness. And your illness may influence the way in which you react to your loved ones.

Close family members can play an important role in providing support and encouragement, but they need to understand the condition in the first place.

Other family members, particularly those that know you less well and who know less about DD, may have simplistic ideas about the condition. Possible reactions are:

- 'Everyone has tummy troubles every now and then, so why make such a fuss?';
- 'If you weren't so stressed your intestines would settle down';
- 'Bowels don't work so well as you get older, so you'll just have to get used to it.'

You can try to explain about DD and give them leaflets, but you may also have to accept that not everyone has the time, patience or sympathy to take on new information. They may have worries of their own.

You may find considerable support and sympathy among your friends, but it may not necessarily be easy for them to understand a disease that shows few external signs and may keep on recurring. On the other hand, having a long-term illness means that those people who continue to be your friends are likely to be good and true friends. Do not forget that friendship is a two-way process and that feeling unwell is not an excuse to avoid putting effort into maintaining and developing friendships.

If your DD is making you reluctant to socialize, you may need to make a conscious effort to meet people. Showing an interest in other people and not worrying too much about your problems is likely to make you more attractive as a friend.

In a marriage, the development of a chronic condition like DD can put a great deal of strain on the relationship. The person with DD might have reduced career opportunities, with financial consequences, or may not be able to contribute much to the housework. Sexual relations may also become more inhibited and less frequent. These stresses and strains may break up the marriage or, alternatively, make it stronger. The difference might lie in the couple's willingness to approach problems that arise, honestly and openly.

In particular, sexual relations may be affected by fears of suffering pain. If you undergo surgery it may take several months before you feel strong enough or confident enough to engage in sexual intercourse. Please remember, however, that sexual love can be expressed by holding and caressing as well as by intercourse, and that it is often the feelings behind the expression of sexual love that are as important as the physical acts. Being able to talk with your partner about sexual worries may not come easily, but it is a good idea to do this to stop a barrier to intimacy undermining the relationship.

Exercise

There is some evidence, described in Chapter 1, that exercise reduces the risk of developing DD. It is not known whether exercise is also helpful once symptoms of DD have started. It is, however, reasonable to make such an assumption. Just as a high-fibre diet reduces symptoms in people with symptomatic DD, as well as protecting people from developing DD, so exercise can be expected to have some benefits in people already diagnosed with DD.

Undertaking increased levels of exercise should be approached with some thought, so that the exercise is active enough for benefits to accrue, but not so vigorous that harm occurs.

Your age and your current level of health and fitness should be taken into consideration when planning greater exercise, and guidance should be sought from your doctor. Your doctor may check your pulse and blood pressure to check if there are likely to be particular risks in exercising. He or she may be able to provide you with an exercise plan. The plan should explain how to become more physically active in a gradual and safe manner that becomes more sustainable for the long term. On

the other hand, gentle exercise, such as walking, can be undertaken by most people without any preparation; so do not delay
just because a comprehensive exercise plan is not yet in place.

If you find the prospect of increased exercise a somewhat
daunting prospect, please bear in mind there are many other
benefits to exercise, such as an improved mental state, strength-
ening of bones, improved cardiovascular condition and
reduction in the risk of developing cancer of the colon.

6

Surgery

There are two types of surgery for DD:

- emergency surgery;
- elective surgery.

Emergency surgery

A small number of people develop very severe abdominal pain and fever without warning. These symptoms develop over several hours and are usually caused by a severe form of diverticulitis, perhaps involving the perforation of a diverticulum, leading to a serious infection within the abdominal cavity. In such cases, the person affected is admitted promptly into hospital. If intravenous antibiotics do not lead to an immediate improvement, the doctor recommends surgery.

If the pain is in the lower-left quarter of the abdomen, acute diverticulitis will be suspected. When someone is feeling very ill, however, some of the usual tests to make a diagnosis are not practical, although a CT scan and an ultrasound may be possible.

The tests may suggest that a diverticulum has perforated, and infection of the lining of the abdominal cavity (peritonitis) may be occurring. Peritonitis is very serious and leads to death in a substantial minority of cases. For this reason, immediate surgery will be recommended, especially if the infection does not respond quickly to intravenous antibiotics. When the patient is told that surgery is needed, in theory he or she can refuse, but when the high risk is explained and the pain is very severe, then few patients, if any, refuse consent.

An operation under such circumstances is called 'emergency surgery' and is undertaken as much to investigate the cause of the severe symptoms as to remedy them. There may not be sufficient time to discuss with the patient all the possible operations for different explanations of the symptoms.

Several studies have shown that less than a quarter of patients who have perforated diverticulitis have had any record of DD symptoms in the past. In other words, most people who have emergency surgery for DD were unaware they had the condition and had little or no forewarning. Consequently, after recovery from emergency surgery, the person may find it difficult, for a while, to come to terms with such a dramatic and unexpected development.

Elective surgery

In most cases of surgery for DD, there is plenty of time to consider and discuss the type of surgery available. This sort of operation is known as 'elective surgery', because the patient has a much bigger say in whether surgery takes place.

Although patients play an active role in making the decision, they will naturally be strongly influenced by the opinion and recommendation of their doctor or surgeon. The difficulty is that there is a vigorous debate among surgeons as to whether and when elective surgery should be undertaken.

Elective surgery as a preventative

Usually, doctors do not recommend surgery after just one episode of diverticulitis, because approximately three-quarters of all such cases never have a recurrence. Many surgeons will, however, recommend surgery after a second bout of diverticulitis. This approach is supported by several authoritative bodies, including the American Society of Colon and Rectal Surgeons, the American College of Gastroenterology and the European Association for Endoscopic Surgery.

These recommendations are given on the grounds that surgery will prevent the development of more serious DD in the future. The thinking is that the greater the number of bouts of diverticulitis, the more difficult it becomes to treat the infection medically (non-surgically). This diminished effectiveness of medical treatment increases the risk that the infection might get out of control, which could then require emergency surgery. It is the development of abscesses that appears to be the main cause of the reduced effectiveness of medical treatment. Although some abscesses resolve, many persist and can be a source of fresh flare-ups of diverticulitis.

The main danger against which elective surgery is meant to protect is peritonitis. Peritonitis requires emergency surgery and the mortality rate for such an operation is greater than for elective surgery. Precise mortality figures are not available for surgery for DD because they vary between hospitals. However, emergency surgery always carries higher risk, at approximately three times the rate for elective surgery. Emergency surgery is also more likely to involve the creation of a colostomy, although this is usually temporary (see 'Surgery details' at the end of this chapter).

Another advantage of elective surgery is that it usually takes place at an early stage in the development of DD. The patient therefore tends to be younger, and younger people usually recover more quickly from surgery.

Critics of the use of elective surgery as a preventative prefer conservative treatment. This is the standard non-surgical approach of antibiotics, liquid diet and bed rest, followed by long-term high-fibre diet. In cases of diverticulitis without complications, conservative treatment is effective in eliminating symptoms in all but a few patients. Critics of elective surgery also argue that evidence is limited for bouts of diverticulitis becoming progressively more severe over time, and point out that elective surgery is not without its risks, particularly for the elderly.

Furthermore, surgery is no guarantee that symptoms will not recur. The statistics show that between 10 and 25 per cent of people continue to experience some symptoms after surgery. In addition, the risk of developing peritonitis in people already diagnosed with DD is considered very small. In a study of 20,000 patients admitted to Washington state hospitals for diverticulitis, but who did not have surgery, only 5.5 per cent required emergency surgery at a later date. More than three-quarters of DD-peritonitis cases occur in people who have never previously had symptoms of DD.

One of the reasons surgeons are disagreeing about elective surgery is that data in some studies are unclear about the classification of recurring symptoms. The symptoms may be from a flare-up of diverticulitis or they may be of the IBS type. While diverticulitis has the potential for causing peritonitis, there is no evidence that IBS-type symptoms risk causing peritonitis.

Recently, some researchers undertook a cost-benefit analysis from the patient's point of view, which concluded that elective surgery undertaken after three bouts of diverticulitis was preferable to that undertaken after one or two bouts. Obviously, this is a generalization; each person's circumstances are unique and surgery should be considered in that context. For example, the presence of complications of diverticulitis is likely to favour undergoing elective surgery, while the presence of other illnesses in addition to DD (making the patient weaker) may weigh against elective surgery.

Elective surgery as a treatment

In addition to elective surgery being used as a preventative against a possible worsening of the condition, it can also be used as a way of dealing with persistent and troublesome symptoms.

The difficulty with this approach is that it is not always clear whether such persistent symptoms are caused by diverticulitis and associated complications or whether they are caused by IBS-type spasmodic responses. This is an important question as the response of the surgeon is likely to differ depending on the source of symptoms.

If the source is diverticulitis, then the surgeon is likely to be sympathetic to undertaking elective surgery. However, diagnosing diverticulitis is not always straightforward. In a study that examined 155 sigmoid colons removed as treatment of diverticulitis, one-third showed no signs of inflammation, although muscle thickening was present. This suggests that those patients without inflammation in their sigmoid colon had severe symptomatic DD rather than diverticulitis, and that it had been difficult for the surgeons to make an accurate diagnosis prior to the operation.

As explained in Chapter 2, accurate diagnosis of diverticulitis may require several tests. Inflammation arising from an infected diverticulum usually remains in the local area and may spread into the surrounding fatty tissues. It will not necessarily spread into the layers of the colonic wall. This means that samples taken by an endoscope from the inner lining of the colon (mucosa) may not show any sign of inflammation when viewed under a microscope, but diverticulitis may still have occurred. The use solely of an endoscope is therefore insufficient in deciding whether diverticulitis is present, and a CT scan is also needed.

It may be that the main source of recurrent intestinal disturbance in people with previous experience of diverticulitis is symptomatic diverticulosis, which has no signs of inflammation and usually provides IBS-type symptoms. DD-associated IBS and standard IBS are very similar, and treatment for standard IBS does not include surgery. Surgeons may therefore be reluctant to operate when there is no evidence of infection and inflammation of diverticula.

Furthermore, several studies have found that people who had surgery for diverticulitis, but were subsequently found to have no inflammation of the diverticula, were more likely to have continuing symptoms than were those who had confirmed diverticulitis.

It is therefore important when considering elective surgery as treatment that patient and doctor have a clear and careful discussion on how to proceed, focusing on the specific characteristics of the patient's history of DD, and clarifying the type of DD and the source of symptoms.

Types of surgery for DD

The aim of surgery for DD is simple. The part of the colon affected by DD is removed, and the two healthy ends of intestine are connected together. There are variations in how this is achieved, but the main purpose of the operation remains the same. There is also a question of whether laparoscopy (key-hole surgery) should be used rather than the standard technique. Details of the different variations in surgery for DD are given at the end of this chapter for those who wish to consider the matter in depth. Information on laparoscopy is included in Chapter 9 on 'Future developments'.

Symptom recurrence after surgery

With the removal of the part of the colon causing trouble, one would think that no further symptoms of DD would be experienced. Unfortunately, between 10 and 25 per cent of people who have had surgery for DD later experience further symptoms.

There are three likely explanations for this:

- symptomatic diverticulosis (IBS-like) was mistaken for diverticulitis;
- diverticula have developed in another part of the large intestine;

- an insufficient length of the colon has been removed.

As explained earlier, surgery for symptomatic diverticulosis is not especially effective in eliminating symptoms, and much less effective than surgery for diverticulitis and its complications. As symptomatic diverticulosis becomes easier to diagnose, it is less likely to be treated by surgery.

In some people who have had surgery for diverticulitis, diverticula may later appear in another part of the colon. It is not clear how common this is or how quickly it might occur. In one study, two-thirds of patients showed no significant increase in the number, size or distribution of the diverticula over a period of five years.

When the sigmoid colon is removed, the lower cut should be in the rectum. This is because the rectum very rarely develops diverticula and therefore there is almost no risk of symptoms developing below this point.

The upper cut should be above the point of colonic muscle thickening. Sometimes there is muscle thickening without diverticula and the surgeon might not remove that section. It may not be realized that not only is colonic muscle thickening a precursor to the development of diverticula, but also that the thickened muscles may play a part in the spasmodic reactions that are involved in IBS-type symptoms. To be confident of removing all current and future causes of DD symptoms, some surgeons remove the whole of the descending colon as well as the sigmoid colon.

To reduce the risk of having recurrent symptoms after surgery, it may be advisable to clarify with your surgeon where the cuts in the colon will be made, and also to maintain a high-fibre diet after recovery from surgery to discourage the development of more diverticula.

Meeting the surgeon

If you decide to have surgery, you will meet a surgeon who will explain the operation to you. If there is anything that is not clear, do ask. This is not always easy; you may not remember the questions you wished to ask or be able to think up new ones in response to the doctor's explanation. Also, senior doctors can appear very busy and you may be reluctant to take up too much of their time. You, however, are the patient of the surgeon who has a duty of care towards you, so do take courage and engage in a conversation. It may be helpful to write down a list of questions beforehand.

Most people appear to be happier the more information they have. This is not true of everyone, however. Details about surgical operations can lead some people to worry more than if they simply put their trust in the skills of the surgeon. Each person is different and such differences need to be respected. If you are a relative or close friend of someone who has DD, you may need to consider whether the person facing the operation really wants a lot of information. It may be that he or she is seeking reassurance from the surgeon, rather than wishing to be given all the details of the operation.

To increase the likelihood that the meeting with the surgeon goes well, you may need to think about what it is the person facing the surgery will be looking for.

If a colostomy is to be formed (see Chapter 7), the patient will also meet a stoma care nurse or a colorectal nurse specialist. The nurse will provide advice and support for managing the colostomy after the operation.

Going into hospital

Before the operation, the hospital will give you written information about what to bring into hospital (such as nightclothes and toiletries), and how to prepare yourself. You will be asked not to eat or drink (except for water) for a period before the operation. Also, you may have to drink a bowel cleanser (bowel preparation), which is a strong laxative, in order to clear out all the remaining faeces (see Chapter 2 on 'Diagnosis and tests').

On being accepted as an inpatient, prior to surgery, a doctor will check your general health. He or she will be looking for any signs of infection or illness (other than DD) that might mean that the surgery would have to be postponed. The information, including temperature, blood pressure and pulse, will also be used as base figures against which your post-operative recovery is measured.

For a colostomy, the stoma care nurse will make a mark on your abdomen where the surgeon will make the stoma. The nurse will discuss with you where the position should be.

You will also be asked to sign a consent form, which provides legal confirmation that you are agreeable to the surgery being performed. The operation will not take place if the form is not signed. If, at the last moment, you decide that you do not want the operation to proceed, you should not sign the consent form. Obviously, it is very disruptive (and costly) for the hospital if you change your mind at the last moment. It is important, therefore, that you give careful thought to the surgery beforehand and are of a firm mind on the matter.

Assuming that you are proceeding with the surgery, an anaesthetist will explain how he or she will make you unconscious and how pain will be controlled after the operation.

Following the operation, you will probably regain consciousness in the recovery room, which is near to the operating theatre. Your condition will be closely monitored, perhaps in a 'high dependency unit' for about two days. Subsequently you will be moved to a room or ward in the hospital where you will recuperate.

To start with, you will have a number of tubes coming out of various parts of your body, either supplying fluids or drugs, or draining urine and bodily secretions. Pain relief will probably be provided by a tube directly into a vein. It may also be provided by an epidural, in which a fine needle is placed in the back. As you recover, you are more likely to have 'patient controlled analgesia' (PCA), whereby you can control the amount of painkiller delivered. There is a safety lock to prevent overdosing.

After a few days you will be allowed to drink water, and food will gradually be reintroduced some days later. Initially the food will be soft, liquid and easily digestible.

The various tubes will gradually be removed, and painkillers may be taken by mouth. You will already be receiving anticoagulant injections to reduce the risk of blood clots, and you will be encouraged to get out of bed and take a walk, even though you may not feel ready to do so.

If you have a colostomy (or an ileostomy), the stoma care nurse will visit you and show you how to look after the stoma (attaching the collection bag and emptying it when full). This may seem a daunting challenge at first, but you will gradually get used to managing it (see Chapter 7 on 'Living with a stoma').

It is not uncommon for people to feel depressed after an operation, perhaps because the body has gone through such a shocking experience. Usually this passes, but if your depression persists, you could seek help from the hospital team responsible for your care. Relatives and friends can also be very supportive. Some hospitals have previous patients willing to visit current patients to share experiences and give encouragement.

Coming out of hospital

The length of stay in hospital depends on the type of operation and how ill you were when you first went in. For most patients their stay in hospital is between 10 and 14 days.

The hospital will give you guidance on what you can do when you return home. You will be advised to avoid heavy work (such as lifting, ironing, vacuuming) until your wounds have healed and you have regained your strength. You may not be able to drive for a month or more and may not return to work for at least a couple of months. The time taken to recover will depend on the type of operation, your age, what type of work you do and your general state of health.

If you have had a Hartmann's procedure (see 'Surgery details' below), there will probably be a second operation to complete the process. This will not take place until you have recovered from the first operation.

For most people, the removal of the part of the colon affected by DD makes them feel a great deal better, because the cause of the symptoms has been removed. For a while, however, you may feel worse, because of the immediate effects of having surgery. You are likely to feel weak and tire easily, and a useful habit could be to rest on your bed for an hour after lunch, to regain strength.

In order to accelerate your recovery, you might want to undertake gentle exercise. Your doctor may be able to suggest a plan for this.

If you have a stoma it will take time for you to get used to it. Talk to and seek guidance from your stoma care nurse. He or she is there to help you.

Conclusion

If you are expecting surgery for your DD, it is hoped that the information here will assist you in conversations with your doctor or surgeon. Also, it is hoped that reassurance has been gained that surgery can be undergone with the minimum of distress. Please remember that a substantial majority of people who undertake such surgery feel very much better.

If you have read the chapter out of curiosity rather than because of any impending surgery, please remember that only a small minority of people with symptoms of DD (less than 5 per cent) will undergo surgery.

Furthermore, it is always advisable to have a high-fibre diet to reduce the risk of DD deteriorating. Doctors in north-east Scotland reported that over a ten-year period, during which time high-fibre diets were introduced for DD patients, there had been a reduction in the percentage of hospital patients requiring surgery. The doctors believed that the high-fibre diet had helped to reduce the need for surgery.

Please also try to keep the use of NSAID and opiate-based painkillers to a minimum, as they appear to be the cause of about one-fifth of all perforations. Further details of this risk are found in Chapter 9 on 'Future developments'.

Surgery details

Resection and primary anastomosis

This procedure consists of removing the diseased segment of the intestine (resection), to be followed by the connection of the two cut ends of the remaining intestine (anastomosis).

This process is completed in one operation (a one-stage procedure) and is usually undertaken in cases of diverticulitis that are without complications. Such non-severe cases are usually treated medically, with antibiotics, but if flare-ups of diverticulitis recur then this surgical procedure will probably be recommended. Increasingly, this procedure is also used in elective surgery for more complicated cases of DD.

A variation on this procedure is to include a protective stoma – Chapter 7, on 'Living with a stoma', is dedicated to this subject.

Hartmann's procedure (resection with sigmoid colostomy and closure of the rectal stump)

This is a two-stage procedure and is most commonly used for emergency treatment of diverticulitis. The first stage involves the resection of the damaged part of the colon. The cut end of the rectum remains in position and is sewn closed so that contents, such as secretions, are not released into the abdomen, but rather will escape through the anus. The other cut end of the intestine (healthy colon) is brought to the surface of the abdomen through the formation of a colostomy (see Chapter 7).

The advantage of the two-stage Hartmann's procedure is that more time is available, between operations, for any infection to be brought under control, before the intestine is reconnected.

After two or three months, the second stage of this procedure takes place, in which the colostomy is closed and the colon is connected to the rectum, so that stool passes through the anus again.

7

Living with a stoma

In some types of surgery for DD, a stoma is formed. A stoma is an artificially created hole on the surface of the body connected to an organ within the body. In surgery for DD, the opening is through the abdomen (tummy). Part of the intestine is brought through the opening and is sewn to the surface of the skin. The contents of the intestine are excreted through the stoma and are collected in a plastic bag that covers the stoma. The stoma therefore acts as an alternative to the anus as a route for excreting faeces.

In most cases, stomas created for people with DD are temporary. The stoma remains for about three months and then is closed by a second operation. Not all stomas, however, are temporary. Some people decide that they do not wish to undergo a second operation to reverse the stoma. In such cases the stoma becomes permanent.

This chapter will describe the different types of stoma. It will also consider what a stoma means in practical and emotional terms.

Types of stoma

The operation to produce a stoma is called an 'ostomy'. If the part of the intestine brought to the outer surface of the abdomen is from the colon, the operation will be known as a colostomy. If the ileum (lower end of the small intestine) is used, then the operation is called an ileostomy. Most stomas in people with DD are formed by a colostomy operation.

Although an ostomy is the process of creating a stoma, the term is also sometimes used to mean the stoma itself, for example, in 'colostomy'. Also, a person who has a stoma is sometimes referred to as an 'ostomate'.

Colostomy

In people with DD, there are two positions on the abdomen where a colostomy is most commonly placed. To gain an image of this, you need to know that when doctors refer to the 'left side' or 'right side' of the body they mean from the patient's point of view.

Left side

With a Hartmann's procedure, the colostomy is usually positioned on the left side of the abdomen, below the level of the navel (belly button). The section of the colon damaged by diverticula is removed and, before the healthy part of the colon is reconnected to the rectum, the healthy colon is brought to the surface to form a stoma. This is known as an 'end stoma', because a completely severed part of the colon (with an open end) is used. The part of the colon that is brought to the surface is the descending (or left-sided) colon and this is why the stoma is formed on the left side.

Right side

The other place where a colostomy may be formed is on the right side, slightly above the navel. This is formed as an addition to a resection and primary anastomosis operation. The stoma is formed to protect the new connection between healthy descending colon and the rectum. The healing of the surgically connected intestine is aided by the absence of faeces, which are diverted away through the stoma. The part of the colon used to form the stoma is the transverse colon, which runs horizontally across the upper abdominal space. The right side of the transverse colon is used in most cases as it is further away from the point of join of the reconnected descending colon and rectum.

The stoma in this case is a 'loop colostomy'. This is because a loop of the colon is brought to the surface through the abdominal hole. A cut is made so that the colon is opened, but the colon is not completely severed. This gives the stoma an external appearance of two tubes, one excreting the faeces and the other leading towards the anus, but not carrying any content. The advantage of a loop stoma is that, on reversal, the sewing of the intestine is less substantial than sewing a fully severed colon to another piece of intestine.

Ileostomy

In some cases, rather than a loop colostomy, a loop ileostomy is formed as a protective ostomy for a resection and primary anastomosis operation. The stoma is usually sited on the right side of the abdomen, below the navel.

A loop ileostomy is smaller than a loop colostomy as the small intestine has a smaller bore than the large intestine. The intestine in an ileostomy protrudes from the surface of the skin by about 2.5 cm, while the intestine of a colostomy is almost level with the abdominal surface. An ileostomy is formed as a protrusion, because the small intestine contains some gut secretions that may irritate the skin. There is less likelihood of leakage onto the skin if the ileostomy protrudes. In the large intestine, many of the irritating secretions are reabsorbed into the body or broken down by gut bacteria, and therefore the contents of the colon are less irritating to skin.

Before the operation

As explained in the previous chapter, emergency surgery will not, by definition, allow much time to discuss the operation let alone the specifics of a stoma. With elective surgery there is time to have such discussions.

If a stoma is to be formed, then a stoma care nurse or gastro-intestinal specialist nurse will visit you and explain what to expect with a stoma. The nurse will also consider where the stoma will be formed. The position of a stoma should be so that:

- you can see it;
- it is accessible in sitting, standing and lying positions;
- it does not get in the way of your usual clothing (for example, a trouser belt);
- it avoids other parts of the body (for example, scars, navel, abdominal fat creases).

The nurse will consider such matters carefully and will recommend a position to you. Although you may not want to think about the prospect of having a stoma, it is important that you take an active interest in where it will be sited so that you are satisfied with its position for practical purposes. The nurse will then put a mark on your abdomen so that the surgeon will know where to form the stoma. The mark will be covered with clear tape so that it is not rubbed away before surgery.

After the operation

After the operation, you will be feeling weak as a consequence of the major shock to the body caused by the surgery. You will also feel drowsy from the after-effects of the anaesthetic. It may also feel peculiar to have various tubes coming out of your body and you may be wondering how large the main wound is on your abdomen. In this weakened and vulnerable state, you will not be at your best when you first see the stoma.

Studies have recorded the feelings of people on first seeing their stoma. They include:

- shock;
- hate;
- disgust;

- repulsion;
- embarrassment;
- devastation;
- unacceptance;
- shame.

Such powerful emotions can lead a person to becoming depressed and withdrawn from communicating with others. The emotions are often especially powerful in people who have had an emergency operation and who were not psychologically prepared for surgery. Even if you have had a discussion with a specialist nurse before the operation there is no real preparation for the sight of part of your intestine on the surface of your body.

Unlike the anus, a stoma has no sphincter muscles. It is, therefore, not possible to control the time when the waste contents are pushed out from the body into the stoma bag. This experience can have a further unsettling effect, because probably you will not have had lack of control over bowel movements since being a baby.

In your darkest moments, please bear in mind that most people gradually come to terms with the stoma and learn how to manage it. If the stoma is temporary, as is the case for most people who have had surgery for DD, it becomes mostly a matter of coping with its practicalities. If the stoma is permanent, then longer-term adjustment is needed.

Many people with a permanent stoma get so accepting of it that they give it an affectionate name, as if the stoma were a friend. In the sense that the stoma has enabled surgery to relieve or eliminate the symptoms, it is a friend. In the case of emergency surgery for peritonitis, the stoma may have saved the person's life.

Practical matters

The stoma will look moist and pinky-red. It looks as if it should be tender, but in fact it has no feeling, as no nerve endings are present on the inner lining of the intestine, which is exposed in a stoma. The stoma can be touched without harm, although as with all openings to the body it is advisable to keep it clean and wash your hands. It may look bigger than you had expected, but its size will subsequently reduce over the following eight weeks or so.

No waste will be produced for a few days after formation of the stoma. Then a semi-liquid content will be excreted. You may notice an unpleasant smell when the bag is changed, but this will reduce when normal foods are consumed. The stoma bag used in hospital will be made of clear plastic so that medical staff are able to observe the stoma and output at any time.

The stoma bag will initially be attached by a nurse, and emptied by the nurse when full. Gradually, as you recover, you will be encouraged to learn how to manage a stoma bag. It fits around the stoma and sticks to the skin. One of the main challenges is to make sure that the opening of the bag is of the right size. It should fit over the stoma sufficiently closely so that there are no leaks. The size of the bag opening can be cut with scissors to fit the size of the stoma (about 2–3 mm wider than the diameter of the stoma). Once the stoma has reduced in size, it should be possible to use bags with a pre-cut opening of a given size to suit your stoma.

There are many variations of stoma bag, and the stoma care nurse will explain the choices. The main difference is between one-piece and two-piece bags. The two-piece bag consists of a part (known as a wafer) that sticks to the skin, and a second piece that is the bag. The wafer has a protruding hard plastic ring, known as a flange. When a two-piece bag is full, the bag is removed, while the wafer remains in place. With a one-piece bag, when the bag needs emptying the whole unit is removed.

Stoma bags are either close-ended or open-ended. Close-ended bags are discarded when full, while open-ended bags are clamped and are emptied without throwing away the bag.

Various accessories go with the stoma bag. There are adhesives that keep the bag in place and skin sealants that protect the skin from the adhesives. There are also barrier pastes (caulking) that make the area smooth around the stoma, to reduce the risk of leaks. You will be guided by the specialist nurse in the use of the accessories, and shown how to clean the skin surrounding the stoma when the bag or wafer has been removed, and how to inspect the stoma.

With a colostomy, the bag is changed usually once or twice a day, depending on how frequent are the muscular contractions forcing the faeces into the bag. The bag is changed when it is a third to a half full. It takes about ten minutes to change. Cleaning the stoma can be the most time-consuming part of the changing procedure.

A colostomy formed from the descending (left-sided) colon produces firm stool, while a colostomy of the transverse colon on the right side will produce much more fluid faeces as the colon has had less time to absorb water into the body. In both cases the bag used will be close-ended. This is because the content is too firm to flow easily out. The bag is detached from the stoma and discarded when full.

With an ileostomy, the bag is emptied about four to six times a day, because of the higher volume excreted compared with a colostomy. The content of an ileostomy bag is of a porridge-like consistency and is emptied into the toilet by undoing a seal (a clip or Velcro) on the bag while it is attached to the abdomen. After two to four days of being emptied, an ileostomy bag should be replaced.

As so much fluid is lost through an ileostomy, it is important that plenty of fluid (10–12 glasses) be drunk daily and extra salt consumed, such as a packet of ready salted crisps a day. People with an ileostomy need to avoid tough foods that might cause a blockage. Signs of blockage are bad-smelling watery output, cramping pains and a distended abdomen, as well as nausea and vomiting.

You may find that all the information about coping with a stoma is too much to take in at once. Furthermore, there may be leakages and spillages from the stoma bag until you get used to it, which can be upsetting. The stoma care nurse is a support and friend, and you should not hesitate to seek his or her help.

Coming out of hospital

On leaving the hospital, you will be given a set of stoma bags – you can choose opaque versions, rather than see-through, if you prefer. Additional stoma bags are by free prescription and can be delivered from a specialist company. A community nurse will visit you at home regularly, until you are confident in coping with the stoma and the wound from the resection has healed.

As you recover, you will start to think about getting out of the house, mixing socially and returning to work. This prospect carries many worries, such as:

- how to conceal the stoma bag under your clothing;
- changing and disposing of the bag when in unfamiliar places;
- controlling gas production and odour from the bag.

These worries may not be as troublesome as you expect. Modern stoma bags, now made of very thin plastic, are not visible under clothes. If you are prepared beforehand, changing a stoma bag can be undertaken smoothly and relatively quickly. Most bags have an opening that releases excess gas, and the filter may contain charcoal, which absorbs smelly chemicals. Odour can also be reduced by avoiding certain foods such as asparagus, beans, cabbage-family vegetables, cheese, eggs, fish, garlic and onions.

Gas in the intestines is caused by swallowed air and by certain gut bacteria. Swallowed air can be reduced by not drinking with straws, chewing gum or smoking. Gas is also released by fizzy drinks and beer. Gas produced by bacteria is reduced by avoiding beans and vegetables of the cabbage family.

Heavy lifting or hard manual work should be avoided as this may put a strain on the intestines and disturb the stoma.

Some of these practical concerns may have been discussed with the stoma care nurse at the hospital, and you could also discuss them with your community nurse. You could also join a patients' organization, such as the Colostomy Association (see Useful addresses). It may boost your confidence to read about others' experiences and to pick up useful tips.

Complications

Sometimes there are problems with a stoma. The most common are a prolapse or a retraction. With a prolapse, the stoma slips forwards so that more of the intestine protrudes from the abdomen. A retraction is the opposite: the stoma slips back into the body. If you see signs of either of these changes, you should inform your stoma care nurse straight away, so that options can be considered.

Another problem can arise when the skin around a stoma becomes sore. This is usually caused by some of the intestinal content leaking out of the bag. Often this is because the bag opening has been cut too large, or has not been reduced in size as the stoma gets smaller in the days after surgery.

Although obstruction is more common with ileostomies, occasionally it occurs with colostomies. This is usually within the first few weeks after surgery, when the intestinal wall is enlarged with extra fluid from bruised tissue.

Permanent stoma

It should be noted that about one-third of people who undergo the first stage of the Hartmann's procedure do not proceed with the second part. This is usually because they are elderly and wish to avoid the worry, discomfort and risk associated with a second operation. This does mean that the colostomy formed in the first stage becomes permanent.

Body image and sexual attractiveness

Most people with stomas believe that they are less attractive sexually, but when partners are interviewed they say that they still find the person with the stoma attractive.

With an end colostomy, but not a loop colostomy, the stoma bag may be replaced for short periods with a stoma cap. This may be more suitable during sexual activity. A stoma cap may also be used during swimming and when playing sport.

Psychological recovery

It is often not easy for the person affected to talk about their stoma as it affects the way that faeces are eliminated from the body. It is also difficult for family and friends to broach the subject directly. It is known, however, that social support is fundamental to a person's adaption to their stoma, so that attending family occasions and getting involved in social activities is worth the effort.

If there are any aspects of a colostomy or ileostomy that are causing you worry or concern, you can discuss them with the stoma care nurse, who is likely to be very helpful and reassuring. Furthermore, additional help is available from the Colostomy Association or the Ileostomy and Internal Pouch Support Group (ia) (see Useful addresses), and there may be a local stoma support group. The manufacturers of stoma products produce useful magazines and information about new products, and more detailed reading is available from books such as *Living with a Stoma* by Dr Craig A. White (see 'Further reading').

Despite various difficulties, most people find they can lead a normal life with a stoma and do not regret the surgery that created it.

8

Special circumstances

There are particular categories of people for whom DD may have distinct characteristics. These categories are:

- people from East Asia;
- the younger patient (under 40);
- the immunocompromised;
- gender.

People from East Asia

In Chapter 1, the difference in rates of DD between Africans and Europeans was considered. It was suggested that this difference could be explained by racial-genetic differences between the two peoples. This idea was rejected on the grounds that the prevalence of DD was growing among urban Africans who had adopted a Western lifestyle and diet.

This conclusion does not mean, however, that genetic differences have no bearing whatsoever on DD within a population. Among people from East Asia, the presence of diverticula in the right-sided (ascending) colon is far more common than among European (Caucasian) people. In East Asians with DD, about two-thirds have their diverticula solely on the right side compared with about 5 per cent of Caucasians with DD.

To what extent is this difference due to genetics and to what extent environment, such as diet? An environmental factor is suggested by a substantial increase in the incidence of DD in East Asia during the second half of the twentieth century.

In the 1960s, DD was almost as rare among people from East Asia as it is among rural Africans. Over the next 40 years, the prevalence of DD increased until it is now found in about one-quarter of all hospital barium enema tests, compared with about 30 per cent of barium enemas in Western countries.

Furthermore, in the Westernized environment of Hawaii, autopsies of Japanese people who had been long-term residents showed that 52 per cent of the large intestines had diverticula. This compares with a figure of 45 per cent in autopsies of Australians. In other words, given a Westernized lifestyle for long enough, East Asian people can develop as high an incidence of DD as Caucasian people.

The most likely explanation for the substantial increase in the numbers of East Asian people with DD is change of diet. In Japan, between 1946 and 1991, the consumption of dietary fibre fell by 42 per cent and the consumption of meat increased about fourfold. Studies in Japan have shown an association between low dietary fibre and a higher incidence of DD. Furthermore, it has been found that DD patients in Taiwan eat significantly more meat than Taiwanese without DD.

In East Asian people with DD, the muscles of the right side of the colon are thickened and the colon forms distinct segments. These changes in the colonic wall are similar to, but not as severe as, those of left-sided DD in Caucasians. Furthermore, studies have shown that East Asians with DD have higher pressure within the right-sided colon compared with those without DD. Also, this right-sided pressure is higher than in the left side of the colon in the same individuals. All these factors point to the cause of DD in East Asian people being similar to that in Caucasians.

If DD is caused by a low-fibre (and possibly a high-meat) diet in both populations, why do the diverticula appear in different parts of colon? It has been suggested by several Japanese and Chinese scientists that the most likely explanation is a racial-genetic factor. Evidence from Hawaii is used to support this explanation. Among Japanese people who have lived in Hawaii for long periods in a Westernized environment, DD is still predominantly right-sided.

What might be the relevant differences between people from East Asia and Caucasians? There is little information about the differences between the large intestines of the two groups. It is known, however, that the sigmoid colon in East Asians is longer and curved differently from the colons of Caucasians. It may be, therefore, that structural differences between the colons of East Asians and Caucasians will be found to explain the different positioning of diverticula.

Although the cause of DD in people from East Asia appears to be the same as among Europeans, there are substantial differences in characteristics of the condition. In addition to the diverticula being predominantly on the right side of the colon, there are fewer diverticula. Usually the numbers are between one and five on the caecum and/or ascending colon. This compares with left-sided DD in Europeans in which diverticula are often counted in tens.

The diverticula on the right side tend to appear at a younger age than for left-sided DD. In addition, right-sided DD affects more males than females, while left-sided DD is slightly more common among females. Over time, there is not much change in the numbers of diverticula, but where this occurs, it tends to be an increase on the right side and on the transverse colon rather than on the left side of the colon.

Symptoms associated with right-sided DD are uncommon. When they occur they are similar to those of left-sided DD, but there are fewer serious complications leading to surgery. The one exception is that the incidence of bleeding tends to be higher and is more likely to require surgery to remedy.

The main problem with right-sided DD is that any pain is usually felt in the lower right of the abdomen, and this pain can easily be confused with several other conditions, especially appendicitis. Pain arising from right-sided diverticula can usually be brought under control by antibiotics. If, however, appendicitis is suspected, then surgery is likely to follow as appendicitis carries with it a high risk of perforation. In other words, although DD in East Asians causes fewer problems than left-sided DD in Caucasians, sometimes surgery may be undertaken unnecessarily because of confusion over the diagnosis. With increased use of CT and ultrasound scans it should be possible to reduce the number of incidents where symptoms from right-sided diverticula are mistaken for appendicitis.

The younger patient (under 40)

Only about 5 per cent of people with diverticulitis are under the age of 40, although there is some evidence that the numbers are increasing as a proportion of all people with DD. In Western countries, the incidence of right-sided DD appears to be slightly higher among younger patients compared to the average for all ages.

Surgery for DD occurs in young people at a higher rate than average. This suggests that such DD is more severe, but the statistics may be misleading. Studies suggest that about a half of young people with diverticulitis have been given surgery because of misdiagnosis. It appears that some doctors misread the symptoms of diverticulitis as signifying more serious complaints, such as peritonitis or acute appendicitis. If a correct diagnosis had been made initially, then surgery might not have been undertaken.

The error in diagnosis of DD in young adults is not so surprising. Abdominal symptoms are difficult to interpret as so many diseases give similar symptoms. Also, as diverticulitis is uncommon among young people it may not be suspected as a diagnosis. The increased use of CT scanners may reduce the uncertainty of diagnosis.

In the case of an accurate diagnosis of DD in a young adult, should the treatment differ from that in older people? There is some controversy about this question. It has been suggested that DD in younger people tends to be more 'virulent'. This means that it is more severe and is more likely to continue to be troublesome than among people in whom DD appeared at an older age. Those doctors who believe this idea are more likely to recommend that surgery be undertaken after one bout of diverticulitis, which is sooner than usually recommended.

The evidence for greater virulence of DD in young adults is conflicting. On balance it seems that there is a slightly higher risk of symptom recurrence among younger people. However, as the average risk of symptom recurrence is low after the first bout of diverticulitis has been successfully treated by antibiotics, the argument for surgery after one bout of diverticulitis seems weak.

It should be remembered, however, that each person is unique, and individual circumstances may mean that surgery for severe diverticulitis is the best course of action. Such issues should be discussed carefully with the doctor or surgeon.

The immunocompromised

The immune system is the body's method of defending itself from potentially harmful germs and chemicals. A person is said to be 'immunocompromised' if their immune system is functioning poorly. People who are immunocompromised are at a higher risk of serious complications from DD, including perforation.

There are two factors in this increased risk:

- low-level symptoms;
- reduced 'walling off' of inflammatory process.

Diverticulitis in the immunocompromised person may produce few symptoms, even when advanced peritonitis occurs.

Therefore, treatment of such a serious infection may be delayed because the patient is not reporting the mild symptoms to their doctor early enough. Furthermore, the immunocompromised body is not so effective in limiting the area that is inflamed. This means that infection can spread and a perforation into the abdominal space becomes more likely.

There are a number of different causes of a person being immunocompromised. These include various illnesses such as HIV/AIDS and those associated with long-term inflammation, such as rheumatoid arthritis, lupus and Crohn's disease. Another source of compromise of the immune system is certain prescribed medicines, which tend to suppress the activity of immune cells and tissues. Such medicines include anti-cancer chemotherapy drugs, steroids, and immunosuppressants such as azathioprine and cyclosporine.

Because of the additional risks associated with DD, immunocompromised patients are likely to have surgery after the first bout of diverticulitis, to remove the diverticula that may perforate. There is also evidence that the immunocompromised patient responds poorly to the usual medical treatment for diverticulitis, and so surgery becomes doubly necessary. Surgery is, however, riskier for people with a weakened immune system, as any subsequent infections are more difficult to overcome. The doctor will, therefore, consider ways in which the immune system can be strengthened before surgery, if at all possible.

For immunocompromised people with a colostomy, there is the additional risk of the yeast candida developing around the stoma, causing a rash. The candida infection can be treated with anti-fungal powder, although sometimes the infection is persistent.

Gender differences

For the most part, DD expresses itself in similar ways in both men and women. There are just a few notable differences. For example, there are more women than men who have DD: about 60 per cent female to 40 per cent male. Female preponderance is reversed in those with DD who are under the age of 40. In this age group, there are about three males to every female.

Healthy women tend to have longer transit times (for the passage of food through the intestinal tract) than healthy men. As a consequence women are more prone to constipation, which may be a factor in the early development of DD. Such slower transit times may therefore be an explanation for the higher incidence of DD in women.

It is not clear, however, why DD should be more common among young men. A tentative suggestion is that female hormones have a protective effect against DD, though they cease to have a beneficial effect after the menopause. This suggestion has not been tested in a scientific study however.

The other major gender difference in DD is found in right-sided disease in people from East Asia. There are approximately two males affected to every female. A firm explanation for this is not available, although the relatively high incidence of right-sided DD in younger adults may be a factor.

9

Future developments

Medical science is continually advancing and it is reasonable to ask what new treatments for DD might be available in the future. This chapter considers the following areas of potential progress:

- painkillers;
- IBS-like symptoms;
- aminosalicylates;
- probiotics;
- laparoscopy (key-hole surgery);
- maternal diet;
- return to a hunter-gatherer diet.

Painkillers

You may be prescribed painkillers for DD or for another condition. Unfortunately, many painkilling drugs have a side effect of disturbing the intestine, including increasing the risk of perforation in people with DD.

There are two main types of painkillers:

- NSAIDs (non-steroidal anti-inflammatory drugs);
- opiates.

NSAIDs are widely-used drugs, especially for osteoarthritis and back pain. They reduce pain, fever and inflammation. There are many different NSAID drugs, including aspirin, ibuprofen and naproxen.

The main side effect of NSAIDs is injury to the mucosal layer of the intestine. This is the inner layer of the intestinal wall and is the part of the intestine that forms a diverticulum. It follows logically that such weakening of the mucosa increases the likelihood that a diverticulum will perforate. Several studies have shown that DD patients who are taking NSAIDs have shown at least double the risk of perforation.

The risk of developing and worsening symptoms from the use of NSAIDs appears to increase if these drugs are taken regularly, although the evidence against aspirin is ambiguous.

An opiate is a drug that contains or is derived from opium, or has opium-like qualities. Although morphine is an opiate, among outpatients it is more common for other opiates, such as codeine and buprenorphine to be prescribed. Other opiates are mixed with paracetamol, such as co-proxamol, co-dydramol and co-codamol.

Evidence points to opiates causing constipation and increasing the pressure within the colonic space. There is also some evidence that suggests opiates increase the risk of perforation in people with DD.

The risk of haemorrhage from diverticula may be increased by another type of painkiller – paracetamol (acetaminophen) – and possibly also from NSAIDs.

Getting the right balance between providing pain relief and not worsening DD symptoms is not easy, as insufficient evidence is available about the level of risk from different painkillers. As knowledge of the effects of such drugs grows with more research, and as new drugs are developed, it will become easier for people to decide how to control pain safely. In the meantime, it may be advisable to keep doses of painkillers to the lowest possible level.

It should be noted that corticosteroid drugs, which are anti-inflammatory, also appear to increase the risk of perforation in people with DD. Steroids should therefore be avoided in people with DD, if possible.

IBS-like symptoms

The symptoms and treatment of people with symptomatic diverticulosis are outlined in Chapter 3. This is an area of considerable debate and a fuller description is included here as future positive developments can be anticipated.

Symptoms arising from diverticula are often caused by diverticulitis (infection and inflammation of diverticula), related complications (such as abscesses) or from haemorrhage (bleeding). However, many people with DD experience symptoms that do not appear to have any of these causes. There are no obvious signs of infection, inflammation or bleeding.

The most common symptom of symptomatic diverticulosis is cramping (spasmodic) pain, most often found in the lower-left area of the abdomen. Other symptoms are bloating and/or flatulence. The symptoms of pain and bloating tend to be worsened by eating food, and relieved by the passage of flatus (gas) or stool, which is often pellet-like. Changed bowel habits, including constipation, occur in some people with symptomatic diverticulosis.

Some doctors believe that all such symptoms are in fact from irritable bowel syndrome (IBS) and that the presence of diverticula is merely a coincidence. Others believe that the symptoms occur because of the presence of diverticula, but that the symptoms are a form of 'irritable bowel' that is hard to distinguish from typical IBS. Evidence supporting this latter view is that standard IBS is most common in younger adults, while diverticular IBS symptoms are usually found in older people. Also, pain in diverticular IBS tends to be in the lower-left abdomen, while standard IBS occurs in various parts of the abdomen.

Disturbed motility

A recent hypothesis for the cause of symptomatic diverticulosis, if proven correct, may offer hope of improved treatment. The hypothesis centres around the motility of the colon in people with DD. Motility refers to the muscular contractions of the large intestine that cause the contents of the colon to move.

Among people with DD, there appears to be a peculiar characteristic concerning the transit time of their colons. Transit time is the time taken for food to pass through the full length of the intestine. Among people with no intestinal disease, the lower the amount of fibre in the diet the slower the movement of the content and the longer the transit time. As people with DD have been shown consistently to have a diet low in fibre, it had been assumed that they would have slow transit times. Three studies have, however, found differently. In those with DD, the transit time was on average quicker than those without DD.

The explanation proposed for this unexpected finding is that people with DD have disturbed patterns of muscle contraction, which in most cases move the gut contents more quickly than average. Most studies of muscles of the colon have shown unusual gut contractions and altered nerve tissue among people with DD. This may lead the colon to go into spasm (a sudden strong muscle contraction).

In other words, people without DD who are eating a low-fibre diet (and perhaps developing diverticula) may have a slow bowel transit time. However, if diverticula and associated symptoms develop, transit time will probably have quickened due to disturbed motility patterns.

How do these abnormal muscle contractions of the large intestine occur? Researchers have looked to IBS for explanations, because IBS causes symptoms similar to those of symptomatic diverticulosis. Furthermore, it has been found that people with IBS and those with DD appear to share a high level of sensitivity to intestinal pain.

The cause of IBS is unknown, but one of many hypotheses is that a gut infection, such as gastroenteritis, stimulates the immune system and this leads to a disturbance of the colon. It is thought inflammatory chemicals that are produced by the body to tackle the gut infection may have the secondary effect of making nerves of the intestine especially sensitive. This may lead to long-term low-level inflammation, through over-reaction to benign bacteria and other mild stimulants. Such inflammation may cause irregular contractions and various associated symptoms.

This possible explanation for the cause of IBS has been adopted for symptomatic diverticulosis by some doctors. It is proposed that IBS-type symptoms develop after the infection and inflammation of a diverticulum. The pain experienced with symptomatic diverticulosis might be ultra-sensitivity to high pressure on the colonic wall, which is typically associated with colonic muscle contractions in people with DD. Sensitivity to spasm of the colonic muscle may also be a factor in the pain of other types DD. Normally, few of the contractions and other movements of the intestine are felt, but this may change if the nerves in the colonic wall become ultra-sensitive.

In support of this hypothesis is evidence that inflammation can occur in and around diverticula without causing noticeable symptoms. In an autopsy study of 90 colons containing diverticula, ten had signs of diverticulitis, but six of the ten patients had not reported any abdominal symptoms. There is also some limited evidence of patients with DD developing IBS-type symptoms following a bout of diverticulitis, although there have not yet been enough studies to be convincing.

If future studies confirm this explanation for symptomatic diverticulosis, then more focused treatments for IBS may be considered. These may include muscle relaxants, such as 'calcium channel blockers', anti-spasmodic drugs, such as dicyclomine, and peppermint oil, which also has anti-spasmodic properties. Furthermore, there may be benefit from anti-inflammatory drugs, such as aminosalicylates, and from probiotics.

Aminosalicylates

As many symptoms of DD are associated with inflammation, then perhaps an anti-inflammatory treatment may prove beneficial. A group of anti-inflammatory drugs, the aminosalicylates, has a long track record of effectiveness in another intestinal complaint, inflammatory bowel disease. One of the aminosalicylates, mesalazine, has been tested on people with DD.

Mesalazine has been found to be effective in lengthening the period when patients are without symptoms. It also reduces the likelihood of bleeding. With a group of 170 outpatients, predominantly with symptomatic DD, mesalazine reduced all symptoms, especially lower abdominal pain, diarrhoea and tenesmus (a feeling of incompletely emptied rectum). Mesalazine was also slightly more effective than a broad spectrum antibiotic.

Furthermore, among a group of 280 patients with a history of recurrent attacks of acute diverticulitis, treatment with mesalazine plus an antibiotic was more effective than antibiotic alone in reducing symptoms and in preventing recurrence of diverticulitis.

More research is needed to confirm these encouraging results. Other anti-inflammatory drugs may prove to be beneficial, and effective dosage levels for different types of DD need to be clarified.

One of the main advantages of mesalazine and similar drugs is that they can be prescribed for a long period without harm, although a few people do experience side effects, such as diarrhoea, nausea and headache.

Probiotics

Probiotics are foods or food supplements, such as drinks, yoghurts and capsules, that contain live beneficial bacteria. They are consumed with the intention of increasing the numbers of such bacteria in the intestine and aiding the functioning of the digestive system. Some probiotics have been shown to be beneficial in cases of infectious diarrhoea and inflammatory bowel disease and they may have a role in DD.

Several studies involving people with symptomatic diverticulosis found that the probiotics reduced or eliminated symptoms and prevented the reappearance of symptoms. In a third study, involving people with recurrent diverticulitis, a probiotic produced significant reductions in symptoms.

More studies will be needed to confirm these early encouraging results. An advantage of probiotics is that they have few if any side effects.

How do probiotics work?

Probiotics appear to work both in people with symptomatic diverticulosis (IBS-like symptoms) and in those with diverticulitis (gut infections and inflammation). How can such a treatment work in both situations? To answer this, it is necessary to understand the bacteria that live in our intestines (known as the microflora or microbiota). There are trillions of these bacteria in each of us, and they have a close relationship with the human body. This relationship has developed over millions of years as humans have evolved. These microflora bacteria protect against infection by pathogens (harmful germs), as well as improving the function of the immune system in the gut wall, and also providing nutrients for the human body.

The beneficial bacteria in probiotic products are usually of species that are found in the human microflora, and they have the potential to bring the microflora back to a healthy balance. Probiotic bacteria can provide benefits in a number of different ways, because they are living creatures that carry with them between two and three thousand genes. They are therefore vastly more complex than a chemical medicine, which will consist of only one or a few molecules.

Certain probiotic strains (variations within a species) are known to reduce IBS symptoms, probably through regularizing gut motility, amending immune function and influencing nerve activity. Other strains will attack infection-causing pathogens, mainly through the secretion of acid and of antibiotic-like molecules. In fact, some strains will be able to work in all these different ways.

It should be noted, however, that as they are living micro-scopic creatures, probiotic bacteria always have the potential to cause an infection themselves, even though this is extremely unlikely. The very slight risk is greater if your immune system is very weak, or if you have recently undergone intestinal or dental surgery. If in doubt, ask your doctor.

Knowledge about probiotic strains is increasing rapidly, and it may soon be possible to purchase products containing strains that have good evidence for treating or preventing diverticular symptoms. In the absence of such a product, a good quality multi-strain product will increase your chances of achieving a positive effect.

At the time of writing, probiotics cannot be prescribed in the UK; and so you will need to pay for them yourself. In time, probiotics will be registered as medicines, and your doctor will be able to prescribe them.

Laparoscopy (key-hole surgery)

Laparoscopy is the use of an endoscope (an optical tube), known as a laparoscope, which is inserted through the abdominal wall to view the organs in the abdomen. Since the early 1990s, the laparoscope has also been used to undertake surgery, such as removal of the gall bladder and removal of a cancerous section of the colon. More recently, laparoscopy has been used in surgery for DD.

When laparoscopy was first introduced it was described as 'key-hole surgery', because the surgeon was able to look into a larger space through a small opening, as a person can look into a room through a traditional key-hole.

The main advantage of laparoscopy is that relatively small incisions are made, compared with the large opening of the abdomen used in standard surgery (open surgery). The small incisions of laparoscopy have the consequence that recovery after the operation is usually much quicker. For example, pain after the operation is usually less, as is the likelihood of developing a wound infection. Also, the time before release from hospital may be reduced from about seven days after the operation to three or four days. Another advantage of laparoscopy is that the size of the scar on the abdomen is much smaller.

Laparoscopy for DD is, however, more difficult than laparoscopy for colonic cancer. This is because the inflammatory process in DD causes the colon to adhere to nearby structures in the abdomen. This makes it difficult to distinguish between the sigmoid colon and other parts of the abdomen and increases the risk that another part of the intestine may be accidentally perforated. With standard surgical methods, it is easier to see the full picture of the abdominal contents and consequently errors are less likely to occur. Also, the greater care needed in laparoscopy for DD means that the operation takes longer to complete than with standard surgery.

It is more likely that surgeons will use laparoscopy for the less complicated surgical cases. Also, a surgeon needs to be skilled and experienced in laparoscopy for other conditions, before undertaking such an operation for DD.

There is a variation of this surgical technique, known as 'hand-assisted laparoscopy', and it has been suggested that it may be more suitable for more complicated cases of DD.

Despite the difficulties of laparoscopy for DD, in the hands of an experienced surgeon it does not appear to be more risky than standard surgery for DD.

It should be noted that in about 10 per cent of all laparoscopy operations it is necessary to change to standard surgery during the operation. This involves making a long incision for a clearer view of the abdomen. In such circumstances, a large scar will be left on the surface of the abdomen.

If you wish to discuss with your doctor the possibility of surgery for DD being undertaken by laparoscopy, please note that the standard way of opening the abdomen for surgery is known as 'laparotomy'. As the two terms sound very similar, you need to make sure you are not confusing them when talking with your doctor.

Maternal diet

Women who are planning to become pregnant may need to ensure that they consume a high-fibre diet prior to conception and during pregnancy. There is some experimental evidence that the diet of mothers affects the tendency of their offspring to develop diverticula.

The relevant study took place in rats. There were three groups of rats. Two of the groups were fed a low-fibre diet, but these two groups differed in that one had been born to mothers who had been on a low-fibre diet and the other to mothers fed on a high-fibre diet. Of the low-fibre rats of low-fibre mothers, 42 per cent developed diverticula after 18 months, and this compared with just 21 per cent of the low-fibre rats of high-fibre mothers. A control group of high-fibre rats of high-fibre mothers developed no diverticula over 18 months.

If the results of this study apply to humans, and this has not yet been confirmed, then a mother on a high-fibre diet during pregnancy may halve the risk of her children developing diverticula during their lives. Obviously, the children would be better off also consuming a high-fibre diet, but a mother cannot control the type of diet her children consume throughout their lives.

The mechanism by which the diet of a mother appears to affect the intestine of her child is not understood, but in time this should be clarified.

Return to a hunter-gatherer diet

Archaeologists are piecing together a picture of the diet of ancient humans. They are achieving this by a variety of means, including examination of human coprolites (fossilized faeces), mummified bodies, and animal and human bones. By these methods, they are able to understand the type of diet consumed as the human body evolved. As this picture becomes clearer, it may be possible to alter one's diet so that it mimics more closely a diet that suits the proper functioning of the human intestine.

Prior to the development of settled populations, for about one and a half million years, humans moved from place to place to obtain fresh sources of food. Such foods were predominantly coarse plant-based foods, such as greens, seeds, stalks, roots and flowers. Some of these foods were ground and cooked. Meat and animal products were also consumed. The meat was initially scavenged from carcases freshly killed by wild animals, but in time humans became hunters and killed their own meat.

Overall, such mixtures of foods consumed by hunter-gatherers contained a much higher amount of fibre compared to the modern diet. Study of modern-day hunter-gatherer populations has found that they rarely have diseases associated with low-fibre diets, including diverticulosis. In other words, a diet that was consumed for one and a half million years by humans has probably influenced the development of the human intestine and the movement away from such a diet appears to cause various diseases.

Perhaps, in the future, dietitians and nutritionists will devise nutritious diets that more closely resemble those consumed by ancient hunter-gatherers and that are practical to follow. Such diets might help make DD disappear as a disease of the modern world.

Useful addresses

The Bladder and Bowel Foundation
SATRA Innovation Park
Rockingham Road
Kettering
Northants NN16 9JH
Tel. (general enquiries): 01536 533255
Helpline: 0845 345 0165
Website: www.bladderandbowelfoundation.org

A national organization for people with bladder and bowel problems, including DD.

The Colostomy Association
Enterprise House
95 London St
Reading
Berkshire RG1 4QA
Tel.: 0118 939 1537
Helpline (24 hours a day): 0800 328 4257
Website: www.colostomyassociation.org.uk

Core
3 St. Andrews Place
London NW1 4LB
Tel.: 020 7486 0341
Website: http://corecharity.org.uk

A national charity supporting research into all diseases of the gut.

The IBS Network (formerly **The Gut Trust**)
Unit 1.16 SOAR Works
14 Knutton Road
Sheffield S5 9NU
Tel.: 0114 272 3253
Website: www.theibsnetwork.org

The national charity for people with iritable bowel syndrome in the UK.

Ileostomy and Internal Pouch Support Group (IA)
Peverill House
1–5 Mill Road
Ballyclare
Co. Antrim BT39 9DR
Northern Ireland
Freephone: 0800 0184 724
Website: www.iasupport.org

Overseas

International Ostomy Association
PO Box 512
Northfield
MN 55057-0512
USA
Toll-free phone: 1-800-826-0826
Website: www.ostomyinternational.org

Organization with branches in various countries.

Further reading

Patricia K. Black and Christine H. Hyde, *Diverticular Disease.* Whurr Publications, London, 2005 (written for health professionals).

Rosemary Nicol, *Coping Successfully with Your Irritable Bowel*. Sheldon Press, London, 1989.

N. S. Painter and D. P. Burkitt, 'Diverticular Disease of the Colon: A Deficiency Disease of Western Civilisation'. *British Medical Journal*, 1971, 2: 450–54.

Craig A. White, *Living with a Stoma*. Sheldon Press, London, 1997.

Stephanie Zinser, *The Good Gut Guide*. Thorsons, London, 2003.

Index